AF212741

Taeniasis and Cycticercosis/ Neurocysticercosis - Global Epidemiology, Pathogenesis, Diagnosis, and Management

Edited by Saeed El-Ashram, Abdulaziz Alouffi, Guillermo Tellez-Isaias, Luís Manuel Madeira de Carvalho and Ebtsam Al-Olayan

Published in London, United Kingdom

Taeniasis and Cycticercosis/Neurocysticercosis - Global Epidemiology, Pathogenesis, Diagnosis, and Management
http://dx.doi.org/10.5772/intechopen.104141
Edited by Saeed El-Ashram, Abdulaziz Alouffi, Guillermo Tellez-Isaias, Luís Manuel Madeira de Carvalho and Ebtsam Al-Olayan

Contributors
Naida Kapo, Jasmin Omeragić, Sabina Šerić-Haračić, Davor Alagić, Seljul M.C. Ramyil, Timothy O. Ogundeko, John Bimba, Cornelius S. Bello, Amos P. Bassi, Anshu Chaudhary, Km Deepika, Bindu Sharma, Hridaya Shanker Singh, Longxian Zhang, Junqiang Li, Hassan Mohammad Tawfeeq, Saeed El-Ashram, Güngör Çağdaş Dinçel, Luís Manuel Madeira de Carvalho, Ebtesam M. Al Olayan, Abdulaziz Alouffi, Beniamino T. Cenci-Goga, Luca Grispoldi, Guillermo Téllez-Isaías, Danielle Graham, Inkar A. Castellanos-Huerta, Víctor Manuel M. Petrone-Garcia, Beniamino T Cenci-Goga, Luís Madeira de Carvalho

© The Editor(s) and the Author(s) 2024
The rights of the editor(s) and the author(s) have been asserted in accordance with the Copyright, Designs and Patents Act 1988. All rights to the book as a whole are reserved by INTECHOPEN LIMITED. The book as a whole (compilation) cannot be reproduced, distributed or used for commercial or non-commercial purposes without INTECHOPEN LIMITED's written permission. Enquiries concerning the use of the book should be directed to INTECHOPEN LIMITED rights and permissions department (permissions@intechopen.com).
Violations are liable to prosecution under the governing Copyright Law.

(cc) BY

Individual chapters of this publication are distributed under the terms of the Creative Commons Attribution 3.0 Unported License which permits commercial use, distribution and reproduction of the individual chapters, provided the original author(s) and source publication are appropriately acknowledged. If so indicated, certain images may not be included under the Creative Commons license. In such cases users will need to obtain permission from the license holder to reproduce the material. More details and guidelines concerning content reuse and adaptation can be found at http://www.intechopen.com/copyright-policy.html.

Notice
Statements and opinions expressed in the chapters are these of the individual contributors and not necessarily those of the editors or publisher. No responsibility is accepted for the accuracy of information contained in the published chapters. The publisher assumes no responsibility for any damage or injury to persons or property arising out of the use of any materials, instructions, methods or ideas contained in the book.

First published in London, United Kingdom, 2024 by IntechOpen
IntechOpen is the global imprint of INTECHOPEN LIMITED, registered in England and Wales, registration number: 11086078, 5 Princes Gate Court, London, SW7 2QJ, United Kingdom
Printed in Croatia

British Library Cataloguing-in-Publication Data
A catalogue record for this book is available from the British Library

Additional hard and PDF copies can be obtained from orders@intechopen.com

Taeniasis and Cycticercosis/Neurocysticercosis - Global Epidemiology, Pathogenesis, Diagnosis, and Management
Edited by Saeed El-Ashram, Abdulaziz Alouffi, Guillermo Tellez-Isaias, Luís Manuel Madeira de Carvalho and Ebtsam Al-Olayan
p. cm.

This title is part of the Infectious Diseases Book Series, Volume 28
Topic: Parasitic Infectious Diseases
Series Editor: Alfonso J. Rodriguez-Morales
Topic Editor: Amidou Samie

Print ISBN 978-1-80356-497-5
Online ISBN 978-1-80356-498-2
eBook (PDF) ISBN 978-1-80356-499-9
ISSN 2631-6188

We are IntechOpen, the world's leading publisher of Open Access books

Built by scientists, for scientists

6,800+
Open access books available

182,000+
International authors and editors

195M+
Downloads

156
Countries delivered to

Our authors are among the
Top 1%
most cited scientists

12.2%
Contributors from top 500 universities

CLARIVATE ANALYTICS BOOK CITATION INDEX INDEXED

WEB OF SCIENCE™

Selection of our books indexed in the Book Citation Index
in Web of Science™ Core Collection (BKCI)

Interested in publishing with us?
Contact book.department@intechopen.com

Numbers displayed above are based on latest data collected.
For more information visit www.intechopen.com

For EU product safety concerns:
IN TECH d.o.o., Prolaz Marije Krucifikse Kozulić 3, 51000 Rijeka, Croatia,
info@intechopen.com or visit our website at intechopen.com.

IntechOpen Book Series
Infectious Diseases
Volume 28

Aims and Scope of the Series

This series will provide a comprehensive overview of recent research trends in various Infectious Diseases (as per the most recent Baltimore classification). Topics will include general overviews of infections, immunopathology, diagnosis, treatment, epidemiology, etiology, and current clinical recommendations for managing infectious diseases. Ongoing issues, recent advances, and future diagnostic approaches and therapeutic strategies will also be discussed. This book series will focus on various aspects and properties of infectious diseases whose deep understanding is essential for safeguarding the human race from losing resources and economies due to pathogens.

Meet the Series Editor

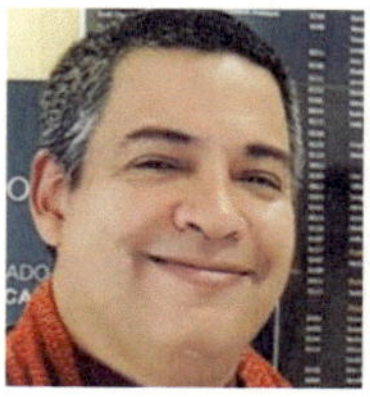

Dr. Rodriguez-Morales is an expert in tropical and emerging diseases, particularly zoonotic and vector-borne diseases (notably arboviral diseases), and more recently COVID-19 and Monkeypox. He is the president of the Publications and Research Committee of the Pan-American Infectious Diseases Association (API), as well as the president of the Colombian Association of Infectious Diseases (ACIN). He is a member of the Committee on Tropical Medicine, Zoonoses, and Travel Medicine of ACIN. Dr. Rodriguez-Morales is a vice-president of the Latin American Society for Travel Medicine (SLAMVI) and a member of the Council of the International Society for Infectious Diseases (ISID). Since 2014, he has been recognized as a senior researcher at the Ministry of Science of Colombia. He is a professor at the Faculty of Medicine of the Fundacion Universitaria Autonoma de las Americas, in Pereira, Risaralda, Colombia, and a professor, Master in Clinical Epidemiology and Biostatistics, at Universidad Científica del Sur, Lima, Peru. He is also a non-resident adjunct faculty member at the Gilbert and Rose-Marie Chagoury School of Medicine, Lebanese American University, Beirut, Lebanon, and an external professor, Master in Research on Tropical Medicine and International Health, at Universitat de Barcelona, Spain. Additionally, an invited professor, Master in Biomedicine, at Universidad Internacional SEK, Quito, Ecuador, and a visiting professor, Master Program of Epidemiology, at Diponegoro University, Indonesia. In 2021 he was awarded the "Raul Isturiz Award" Medal of the API and, the same year, the "Jose Felix Patiño" Asclepius Staff Medal of the Colombian Medical College due to his scientific contributions to the topic of COVID-19 during the pandemic. He is currently the Editor in Chief of the journal Travel Medicine and Infectious Diseases. His Scopus H index is 55 (Google Scholar H index 77) with a total of 725 publications indexed in Scopus.

Meet the Volume Editors

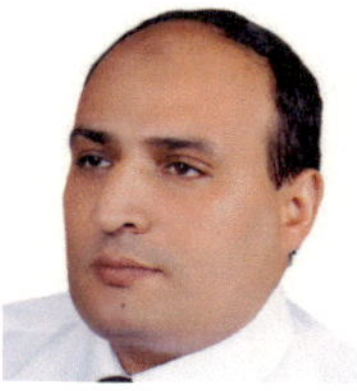

Doctor Saeed El-Ashram is a professor at Kafrelsheikh University, Egypt, and Foshan University, China, and a research professor at Zhaoqing Dahuanong Biology Medicine Co., Ltd., China. His primary research focus is to understand how the animal immune system recognizes and responds to parasitic infections with and/or without a microbial community. Some of these infections, such as toxoplasmosis, cryptosporidiosis, alveolar echinococcosis, and fascioliasis, cause significant diseases in humans, while others, including cryptosporidiosis and coccidiosis, represent a substantial financial burden for food producers. Dr. El-Ashram has more than 120 journal publications to his credit, holds several registered patents, and is an academic editor and reviewer.

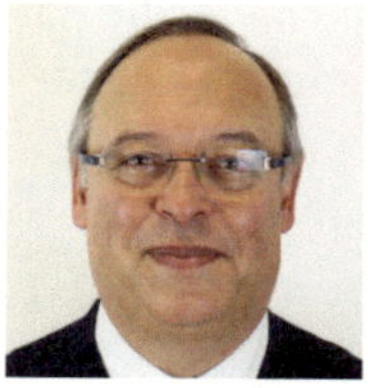

Doctor Luís Manuel Madeira de Carvalho is a Full Professor of Parasitology, Parasitic and Wildlife Diseases at the Integrated Master of Veterinary Medicine (MIMV), Faculty of Veterinary Medicine, University of Lisbon, Portugal. His main areas of interest in teaching and research focus on helminths of domestic animals, exotic pets, and wildlife, namely concerning gastrointestinal and vector-borne parasites as zoonotic agents, interconnected with ecosystem health and conservation medicine. He has more than 200 scientific publications to his credit and has coordinated and/or collaborated in more than 30 research projects concerning parasitology of domestic animals and wildlife. He has supervised around 180 graduate works, including intern and undergraduate reports, master's dissertations, Ph.D. theses, and training at the Parasitology and Parasitological Diseases Laboratory. He is also a reviewer of several international journals.

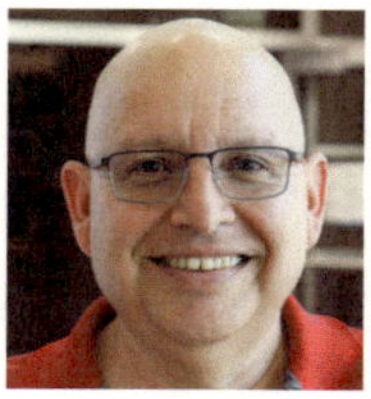

Guillermo Tellez-Isaias received his MS and DVM in Veterinary Sciences from the National Autonomous University of Mexico (UNAM), and his Ph.D. from Texas A&M University, USA. He worked as a professor at UNAM for 16 years, 8 as head of the Avian Medicine Department, College of Veterinary Medicine. Dr. Tellez-Isaias was president of the National Poultry Science Association of Mexico, and a member of the Mexican Veterinary Academy and the Mexican National Research System. Currently, he is a research professor at the Center of Excellence in Poultry Science, University of Arkansas, USA. His research is focused on poultry gastrointestinal models to evaluate the beneficial effects of functional foods to enhance intestinal health and disease resistance.

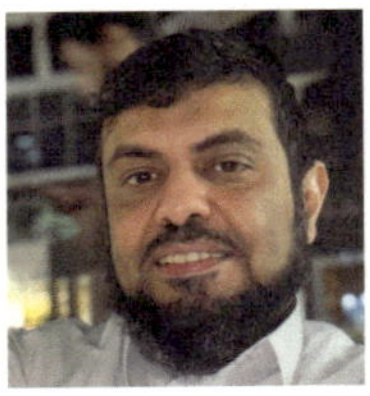

Abdulaziz Alouffi is an associate research professor at King Abdulaziz City for Science and Technology (KACST), Saudi Arabia. He obtained a DVM from Qassim University, Saudi Arabia, and a Ph.D. from the University of Nottingham, UK, with a thesis focused on understanding the roles of Immunoglobulin E (IgE) in human resistance to infection with metazoan parasites (e.g., *Schistosoma spp.*) and how this knowledge can be exploited for vaccination. Currently, Dr. Alouffi is working on zoonoses, using different diagnostic methods, such as a metagenomics approach, to identify zoonotic diseases. In addition, he is using technology to find new targets for the development of more efficient vaccines against zoonotic disease.

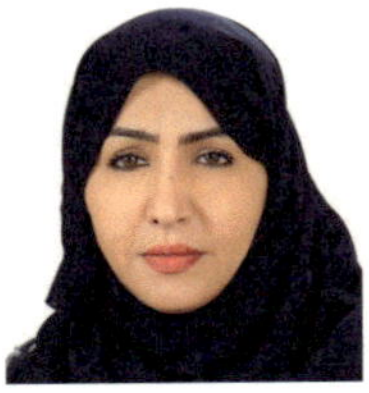

Doctor Ebtsam Al-Olayan is a Professor of Parasitology at the Department College of Science, King Saud University, Saudi Arabia. She is also a supervisor of Chair Vaccines Research of Infectious Diseases, at King Saud University. Dr. Al-olayan has been involved in research of parasitic diseases and vaccines. She has received several awards and is an academic reviewer for many journals. She has registered several patents and has more than eighty-eight publications to her credit.

Contents

Preface

Taeniasis and cysticercosis are two closely related parasitic diseases caused by the tapeworm *Taenia solium*. Taeniasis is an intestinal infection with the adult tapeworm, while cysticercosis is a tissue infection with the larval stage of the tapeworm. Neurocysticercosis is a particularly serious form of cysticercosis that affects the nervous system. Humans are known hosts for two well-known *Taenia* species: *T. saginata* (the cattle tapeworm) and *T. solium* (the pig tapeworm). *T. asiatica*, a third species that shares traits with the other two because its adult morphology resembles that of *T. saginata* and its life cycle corresponds to that of *T. solium*, was identified in the 1990s.

Cysticercosis is caused by *T. solium* and *T. saginata* larva (cysticercus) and manifests itself in the host's internal organs, pigs and cattle, respectively. Neurocysticercosis results from *T. solium* cysticercus infection of the host's central nervous system, namely humans with accidental larval infection. Taeniasis and cysticercosis are major public health problems in many parts of the world, particularly in developing countries. Taeniasis is estimated to affect more than 200 million people worldwide, and cysticercosis affects more than 50 million people. Neurocysticercosis is a leading cause of epilepsy in developing countries. This book provides a comprehensive overview of taeniasis and cysticercosis, focusing on the latest advances in epidemiology, diagnosis, treatment, and control. The book includes seven chapters.

Chapter 1: "Introductory Chapter: Taeniasis and Cysticercosis/Neurocysticercosis – Differences, Risk Factors, and Vaccines"

Chapter 2: "Epidemiology of Taeniosis/Cysticercosis in Humans and Animals"

Chapter 3: "The Pandemonium of Cysticercosis in Humans"

Chapter 4: "*Taenia solium* Taeniasis and Cysticercosis Prevalence and Control Practice in China"

Chapter 5: "Neurocysticercosis: A Review on Global Neurological Disease"

Chapter 6: "Advances in the Diagnosis of Cysticercosis"

Chapter 7: "Neurocysticercosis: An Overview of Pathology and Pathogenesis"

This book is intended for many readers, including researchers, clinicians, public health professionals, and students. It is written in a clear and concise style and includes a wealth of up-to-date information on taeniasis and cysticercosis. It is also intended to raise awareness of these two important diseases and to promote the development of new and improved strategies for their prevention and control. This book covers specific topics on the two *Taenia* species that infect humans, *T. solium* and *T. saginata*, and a third species, *T. asiatica*. It also covers the epidemiology of taeniasis and cysticercosis in humans and animals and the pandemonium of cysticercosis in humans. The book also discusses the prevalence and control of *T. solium* taeniasis and cysticercosis in China and neurocysticercosis as a global major cause of neurological disease. Finally, the book examines advances in the diagnosis of cysticercosis and provides an overview of the pathology and pathogenesis of neurocysticercosis.

I am especially grateful to the authors for sharing their expertise and knowledge on this important topic. Their contributions are invaluable and will help to raise awareness of taeniasis and cysticercosis and promote the development of new and improved prevention and control strategies.

I would like to express my sincere gratitude to Senior Commissioning Editor Lucija Tomicic-Dromgool and Publishing Process Manager – Product Lead Marica Novakovic at IntechOpen. I am also truly grateful to the entire publishing and production team for their hard work and dedication to this book.

Thank you again to everyone who has contributed to this book. Your hard work and dedication are greatly appreciated.

Saeed El-Ashram
Faculty of Science,
Zoology Department,
Kafrelsheikh University,
Kafr El-Sheikh, Egypt

College of Life Science and Engineering,
Foshan University,
Foshan, China

Luís Manuel Madeira de Carvalho
Parasitology and Parasitological Diseases Laboratory,
CIISA – Center for Interdisciplinary Research in Animal Health,
Faculty of Veterinary Medicine,
University of Lisbon,
Lisbon, Portugal

Associated Laboratory for Animal and Veterinary Science (AL4AnimalS),
Lisbon, Portugal

Dr. Guillermo Tellez-Isaias
Division of Agriculture,
Department of Poultry Science,
University of Arkansas,
Fayetteville, AR, USA

Abdulaziz Alouffi
Associate Professor of Infectious Diseases (Zoonotic Diseases) and Vaccinology,
King Abdulaziz City for Science and Technology,
Riyadh, Saudi Arabia

Dr. Ebtsam Al-Olayan
Department of Zoology,
College of Science,
King Saud University,
Riyadh, Saudi Arabia

Chapter 1

Introductory Chapter: Taeniasis and Cysticercosis/ Neurocysticercosis – Differences, Risk Factors, and Vaccines

Güngör Çağdaş Dinçel, Luís Manuel Madeira de Carvalho, Ebtsam Al-Olayan, Abdulaziz Alouffi, Beniamino T. Cenci-Goga, Luca Grispoldi, Guillermo Tellez-Isaias, Danielle Graham, Inkar A. Castellanos-Huerta, Victor M. Petrone-Garcia and Saeed El-Ashram

1. Introduction

Humans are known hosts for two well-known *Taenia* species: *Taenia saginata* (the cattle tapeworm) and *Taenia solium* (the pig tapeworm). *Taenia asiatica*, a third species that shares traits with the other two because its adult morphology resembles that of *T. saginata*, and its life cycle corresponds to that of *T. solium*, was identified in the 1990s. Cysticercosis is caused by the *T. solium* and *T. saginata* larva (cysticercus) and manifests itself in the host's internal organs, pigs and cattle, respectively; neurocysticercosis (NCC) results from *T. solium* cysticercus infection of the host's central nervous system, namely humans with larval accidental infection [1].

2. *Taenia* life cycles

Figure 1 depicts the human *Taenia* spp. life cycle. *T. asiatica* and *T. solium* use the pig as an intermediate host (IH), while *Taenia saginata* uses cattle as an IH. In the small intestine of intermediate hosts, the enveloping structures of taeniid eggs undergo digestion. Subsequently, the oncospheres enter the host's circulation, eventually navigating to their intended target organs via the intestinal membrane. When humans accidentally consume these eggs, namely those of *T. solium*, they can encyst in various tissues (cysticercosis), with a particular affinity for the brain, resulting in NCC. The clinical features of NCC vary depending on the parasites' location, quantity, maturation, regression phases, and the host's immunological response.

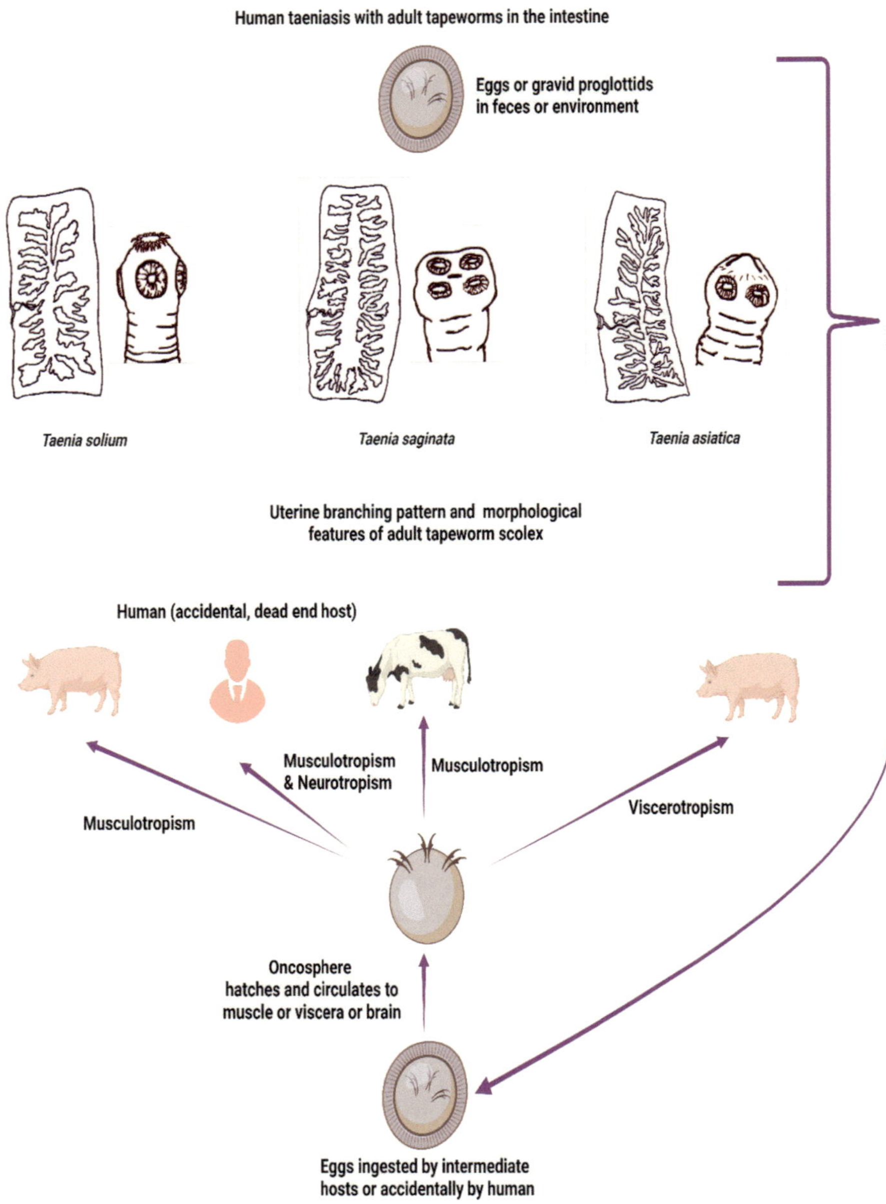

Figure 1.
T. saginata, T. asiatica, and T. solium life cycles.

The scolex of the parasite will evaginate and attach to the mucosa of the duodenum-jejunum if an individual eats uncooked or semi-cooked pork or beef with live cysticerci. Gravid proglottids are passed naturally or via bowel movements 8–12 weeks after infection. Eggs consumed by pigs or cattle are broken down into their embryophoric structures, and the oncospheral membrane is digested by bile and enzymes. It takes around 12 weeks for cysticerci to develop in a pig's skeletal muscle, heart muscle, and brain. These cysticerci will continue reproducing until the pigs are slaughtered for at least a year. *T. saginata* cysticercus has a limited life history, as shown by the calcification of its cysticerci in mature cattle. The cysticerci of *T. saginata* and *T. asiatica* vary primarily because the former are musculotropic in cattle (especially in the liver), while the latter are viscerotropic in pigs. About 8–10 weeks after infection, metacestodes from cattle and swine become infectious to humans. Eggs from infected *T. solium* adults may spread the disease to humans when ingested via the fecal-oral pathway (**Table 1**).

Morphological features	***T. solium***	***T. saginata***	***T. asiatica***
Mature proglottid			
Testis (number)	375–575	800–1200	324–1216
Ovary (number of lobes)	3	2	2
Vaginal sphincter	—	+	+
Gravid proglottid			
Uterine branches (each side number)	7–16	14–32	11–31
Pattern of uterine branching	Dendritic	Dichotomous	Dichotomous
Posterior protuberance	—	+	+
Size (length × width; mm)	3.1–10 × 3.8–8.7	10–20 × 6.5–9.5, longer than wide	4–22 × 3–12
Scolex			
Shape	Globular	Quadrilateral	Quadrilateral
Rostellum	+	—	+
Number of hooks	22–32	—	—
Diameter (mm)	0.6–1.0	1.5–2.0	0.8
Adult tapeworm			
Length (m)	1–5	4–12	1–8
Number of proglottids	700–1000	1000–1500	200–1200
Oncosphere			
Tissue tropism	Musculotropism and neurotropism	Musculotropism	Viscerotropism
Cysticercosis/neurocysticercosis	*Cysticercus cellulosae* in pork	Metacestode, *Cysticercus bovis* in cattle	Metacestode, *Cysticercus viscerotropica* in pig
Cysticercus			
Size (mm)	5–8 × 3–6	6–10 × 4–6	2 × 2
Hooks in scolex	+	—	Rudimentary
Genomic features			
Assembly size (Mb)	131	169	168
GC content (%)	43.5	43.5	43.2
Coding gene number	11,902	13,161	13,323
Average gene length (Kb)	4.6	6.0	5.9
Protein length (aa)	444	464	466
Gene density (genes per Mb)	90.9	77.9	79.3

Morphological features	*T. solium*	*T. saginata*	*T. asiatica*
No. of exons/gene	6.6	6.2	6.2
Exon mean length (bp)	237	237	244
Intron no./gene	5.6	5.2	5.2
Intron mean length (bp)	775	864	831
Exon GC content (%)	50.2	49.7	49.6
Intron GC content (%)	40.8	41.5	41.2
Repeat content (%)	18.1	10.4	10.9
tRNA number	162	339	353

+ Present; – absent.

Table 1.
T. saginata, T. asiatica, and T. solium morphological and genetic differences [2–4].

3. *Taenia* egg survival and dispersal

Taeniid eggs can survive for up to a year in moderate temperatures and are commonly found on vegetables, soil, and water samples, posing a risk to consumers. Invertebrates may serve as transport hosts for taeniid eggs, and wastewater treatment systems are not completely effective in removing them, making access to surface water and using sewage sludge as pasture fertilizer significant risk factors for bovine cysticercosis [5, 6]. However, flies and dung beetles play no significant role in transmitting *T. solium* to pigs, and corralling reduces but does not eliminate

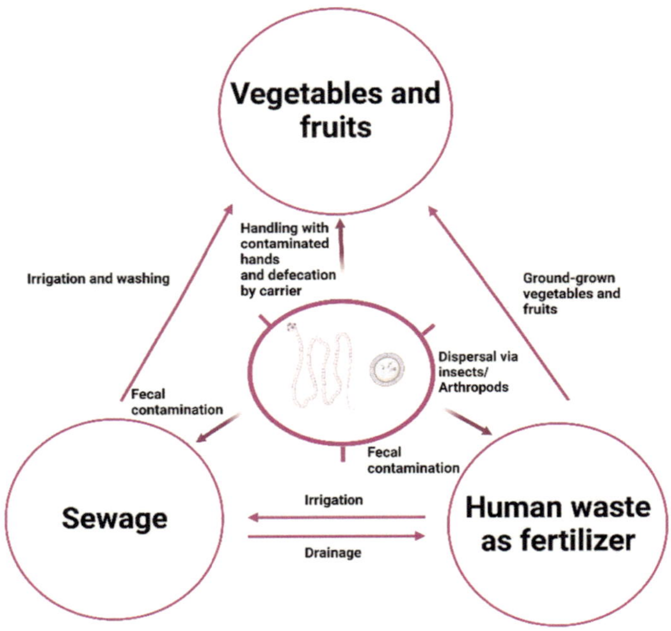

Figure 2.
Taeniid eggs in a variety of environmental matrices [7].

the infection risk with cysticercosis (**Figure 2**). Other mechanisms of egg dispersal should be evaluated for a better understanding of transmission dynamics [8].

4. Risk factors for bovine cysticercosis (BCC)

Bovine cysticercosis is a disease that affects cattle and is caused by a parasite called *T. saginata.* Identified risk factors include herd/farm-related, feed-related, and animal-related factors. Age and gender of animals are correlated with the occurrence of bovine cysticercosis. Environmental contamination is the main cause of BCC cases (**Figure 3**).

5. Risk factors for porcine cysticercosis

Pigs may get infected with *T. solium* or *T. asiatica* if they consume eggs shed by human tapeworm carriers. Although both parasites harm humans, only *T. solium* causes neurocysticercosis, a serious public health problem worldwide. Furthermore, both parasites have an economic influence on the livestock sector. *T. solium* and *T. asiatica* have the same transmission paths from humans to pigs and back. Site transmission may therefore be addressed using comparable intervention strategies. Cysticercosis can be caused by *T. solium* in both humans and pigs. The major cysticercosis risk factor is the presence of adult *T. solium* in human carriers. The main

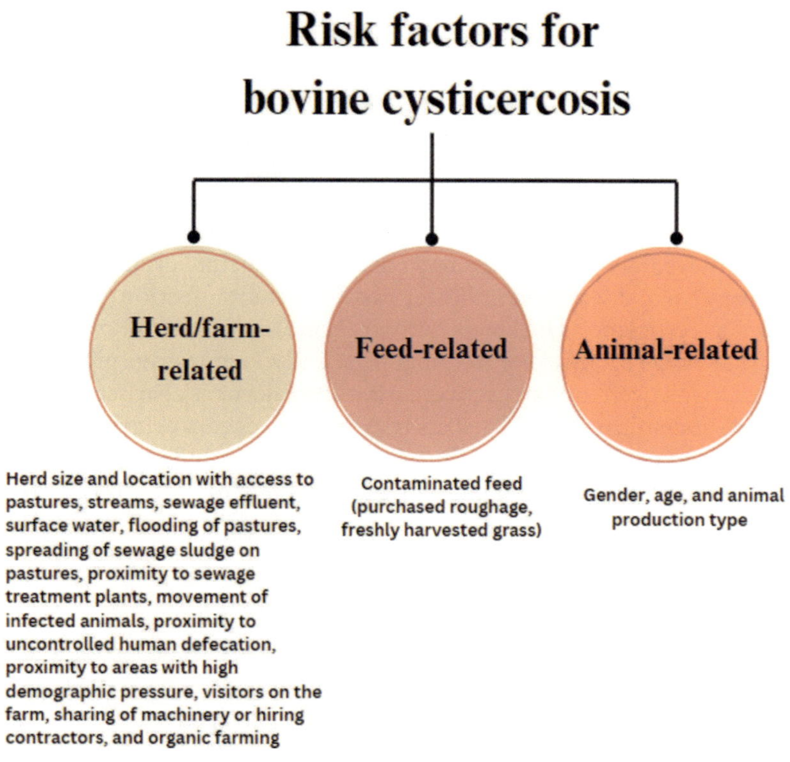

Figure 3.
Risk factors for bovine cysticercosis [9–13].

risk factor for humans getting adult *T. solium* is the inclusion of contaminated pork in the food chain. Free-range pig rearing and the absence or incorrect use of latrines are other *T. solium* cysticercosis risk factors in pigs. These risk factors are prevalent in many low-income Latin American, Asian, and sub-Saharan African countries. Increased age, feedstuff, and dirt floors have also been identified as *T. solium* cysticercosis risk factors in pigs [14–18]. In endemic areas with improper use or a lack of latrines, causing public defecation, roaming pigs are more likely to contract *T. solium* cysticercosis. Low-income endemic regions with free-roaming pigs, indiscriminate feces contamination, and poor personal and meat hygiene, inadequate or nonexistent meat inspection, are particularly susceptible to *T. solium* infection. These risk factors are strongly associated with illiteracy, choices in life, and poverty. In addition, milder infections are typically brought on by indirect transmission, while heavier infections are typically brought on by infective egg direct ingestion produced by *Taenia* carriers. Although we emphasize the seriousness of severe infections, we propose that moderate infections pose a hidden risk and a distinct public health concern because it is more possible that both pre- and postmortem examinations will miss them, allowing them to enter the food chain and pose a public health risk [19].

6. Risk factors for human taeniasis and cysticercosis

One of the risk factors is eating undercooked pork, which can contain the larvae of the tapeworms. Another risk factor is living in a household with infected pigs. Pigs can act as intermediate hosts for the tapeworms, and their meat can be contaminated with the larvae. In addition, humans can shed tapeworm eggs in their feces, which can contaminate the environment and infect both pigs and humans. The risk of infection is higher in females aged 10–39 years, although the reasons for this are not clear. It could be due to differences in dietary habits, hygiene practices, or hormonal factors. The presence of *Taenia* carriers in the household is also a risk factor. These are individuals who are infected with tapeworms and can shed their eggs in their feces, contaminating the environment and infecting others. Seropositivity for anti-cysticercus antibodies is a risk factor. This means that the person has been exposed to the tapeworm larvae and has developed an immune response against them. Seropositivity can be detected through blood tests and indicates past or current infection [20–24]. Risk factors for porcine cysticercosis include a human *Taenia* carrier existence, the absence of a latrine, a free-range backyard or roaming pigs, and a seropositive pig with a *Taenia* carrier nearby. However, human cysticercosis outbreaks have also been reported in urban areas of endemic nations. *T. solium* transmission occurs primarily in rural areas of underdeveloped nations with significant pig ownership, but human cysticercosis outbreaks have also been reported in urban areas of endemic nations [25, 26].

7. Livestock cysticercosis vaccinations

Researchers have developed subunit vaccines against echinococcosis and cysticercosis based on ovine and bovine protective immune responses after egg challenge or immunization with taeniid oncosphere antigen extracts. In 1989, the first recombinant subunit anti-parasite vaccine (To45W) was generated to fight *Taenia ovis* infections, a nonzoonotic metacestode disease of economic relevance in sheep. Bovine cysticercosis-causing *T. saginata* was found to contain homologous genes, and when the produced peptides (TSA-9/TSA-18) were administered intramuscularly to calves with adjuvant, 99% protection was seen against oral challenge with *T. saginata* eggs. This means that the vaccination effectively protected the calves from the disease caused by *T. saginata*. Further efforts have been focused on scaling up the manufacturing of ovine and bovine cysticercosis vaccines so that sufficient quantities and quality-controlled vaccinations are accessible for practical usage. Pigs were also protected against experimental egg challenge infection by a *T. solium* recombinant subunit oncosphere vaccine (TSOL18) for cysticercosis, the most efficient protective vaccination in pigs against *T. solium* cysticercosis [27]. The researchers have focused on scaling up the manufacturing of both vaccines to make them more accessible for practical usage. The study found that pigs were protected against experimental egg challenge infection by a *T. solium* recombinant subunit oncosphere vaccine (TSOL18) for cysticercosis. TSOL18 is the most efficient protective vaccination in pigs against *T. solium* cysticercosis, which makes it a promising candidate for further studies and inclusion in *T. solium* control programs [28–30]. In mice, the expression and immunogenicity of the codon-optimized TSOL18 gene were much higher than those of the un-optimized gene. These findings provide the groundwork for developing an improved TSOL18 gene vaccination against cysticercosis [31]. The TSOL16 antigen (for ovine psoroptic mange control) might be a beneficial addition to existing swine vaccination approaches, allowing for the development of novel *T. solium* cysticercosis vaccine tactics [32]. With oral vaccination, the recombinant pMG36e-SP-TSOL18/*Lactococcus lactis* and pMG36e-TSOL18/*L. lactis* vaccines can trigger specific mucosal, cellular, and humoral immunity in mice. More notably, the recombinant pMG36e-SP-TSOL18/*L. lactis* vaccination produces a stronger immunological response, which reveals the feasibility of employing the *L. lactis* strain as a vehicle to carry *T. solium* protective antigens [33]. Although there have been discussions about the therapeutic immunization of intermediate hosts against *Taenia* larval cysts, it remains in its nascent phases, and more research is needed to develop effective therapies.

8. Conclusion

A standardized detection instrument is needed to understand the epidemiology of *Taenia* species and develop strategies for enhancing veterinary public health. Vaccinating swine with recombinant *T. solium* antigens and anthelmintics may reduce the risk of infection in human populations in endemic areas. Moreover, a comprehensive One Health approach, including interventions for people, pigs, and the environment, is expected to result in a stronger and longer-lasting benefit in eliminating cysticercosis.

Acknowledgement

The authors extend their appreciation to the Deanship of Scientific Research, Kind Saud University for funding Through Vice Deanship of Scientific Research Chairs, Research Chair of Vaccine against infectious Diseases.

Author details

Güngör Çağdaş Dinçel[1], Luís Manuel Madeira de Carvalho[2,3], Ebtsam Al-Olayan[4], Abdulaziz Alouffi[5], Beniamino T. Cenci-Goga[6], Luca Grispoldi[6], Guillermo Tellez-Isaias[7], Danielle Graham[7], Inkar A. Castellanos-Huerta[7], Victor M. Petrone-Garcia[8] and Saeed El-Ashram[9,10]*

1 Eskil Vocational School, Laboratory and Veterinary Science, Aksaray University, Aksaray, Turkey

2 Parasitology and Parasitological Diseases Laboratory, CIISA – Center for Interdisciplinary Research in Animal Health, Faculty of Veterinary Medicine, University of Lisbon, Lisbon, Portugal

3 Associated Laboratory for Animal and Veterinary Science (AL4AnimalS), Lisbon, Portugal

4 Department of Zoology, College of Science, King Saud University, Riyadh, Saudi Arabia

5 Associate Professor of Infectious Diseases (Zoonotic Diseases) and Vaccinology, King Abdulaziz City for Science and Technology, Riyadh, Saudi Arabia

6 Food Safety and Inspection, Department of Veterinary Medicine, University of Perugia, Italy

7 Division of Agriculture, Department of Poultry Science, University of Arkansas, Fayetteville, AR, USA

8 Departamento de Ciencias Pecuarias, Universidad Nacional Autónoma de México (UNAM), Cuautitlan Izcalli, México

9 Faculty of Science, Zoology Department, Kafrelsheikh University, Kafr El-Sheikh, Egypt

10 College of Life Science and Engineering, Foshan University, Foshan, China

*Address all correspondence to: saeed_elashram@yahoo.com

IntechOpen

© 2023 The Author(s). Licensee IntechOpen. This chapter is distributed under the terms of the Creative Commons Attribution License (http://creativecommons.org/licenses/by/3.0), which permits unrestricted use, distribution, and reproduction in any medium, provided the original work is properly cited.

References

[1] Galán-Puchades MT, Fuentes MV. Lights and shadows of the *Taenia asiatica* life cycle and pathogenicity. Tropical Parasitology. 2013;**3**(2):114-119

[2] Wang S, Wang S, Luo Y, Xiao L, Luo X, et al. Comparative genomics reveals adaptive evolution of Asian tapeworm in switching to a new intermediate host. Nature Communications. 2016;**7**:12845

[3] Flisser A. State of the art of *Taenia solium* as compared to *Taenia asiatica*. The Korean Journal of Parasitology. 2013;**51**(1):43-49

[4] Victor B. Proteomic analysis of *Taenia* spp. excretion/secretion proteins: the search for *Taenia solium*-specific diagnostic antigens; 2014

[5] Jansen F et al. The survival and dispersal of *Taenia* eggs in the environment: what are the implications for transmission? A systematic review. Parasites & Vectors. 2021;**14**(1):88

[6] Malkamäki S et al. Dispersal of taeniid eggs: Experimental faecal contamination of forest environment followed by DNA detection in wild berries. Food and Waterborne Parasitology. 2022;**27**:e00152

[7] Saelens G, Robertson L, Gabriël S. Diagnostic tools for the detection of taeniid eggs in different environmental matrices: A systematic review. Food and Waterborne Parasitology. 2022;**26**:e00145

[8] Gonzales-Gustavson E et al. Evaluating the role of corrals and insects in the transmission of porcine cysticercosis: A cohort study. Pathogens. 2023;**12**(4):597

[9] Blagojevic B et al. Bovine cysticercosis in the European Union: Impact and current regulations, and an approach towards risk-based control. Food Control. 2017;**78**:64-71

[10] Samorek-Pieróg M, Karamon J, Cencek T. Identification and control of sources of *Taenia solium* infection - the attempts to eradicate the parasite. Journal of Veterinary Research. 2018;**62**(1):27-34

[11] Macrelli M et al. Bovine cysticercosis outbreak in an indoor beef finisher farm in the North of England. Veterinary Record Case Reports. 2020;**8**(3):e001178

[12] Dixon MA et al. *Taenia solium* taeniasis/cysticercosis: From parasite biology and immunology to diagnosis and control. Advances in Parasitology. 2021;**112**:133-217

[13] Mendlovic F, Fleury A, Flisser A. Zoonotic *Taenia* infections with focus on cysticercosis due to *Taenia solium* in swine and humans. Research in Veterinary Science. 2021;**134**:69-77

[14] Thomas LF et al. Prevalence of *Taenia solium* cysticercosis in pigs entering the food chain in western Kenya. Tropical Animal Health and Production. 2016;**48**(1):233-238

[15] Chaisiri K et al. Gastrointestinal helminths and *Taenia* spp. in parenteral tissues of free-roaming pigs (*Sus scrofa indicus*) from hilltribe village at the western border of Thailand. Tropical Biomedicine. 2017;**34**(2):464-470

[16] Oleleu A-M et al. Seroprevalence of porcine cysticercosis and influence of some associated risk factors in Northwestern Romania. Acta Veterinaria Brno. 2016;**85**:121-126

[17] Nguyen TTM et al. Occurrence of *Taenia* species in pigs in slaughterhouses in Phu Tho province, northern Vietnam. Journal of Helminthology. 2020;**94**:e201

[18] Trevisan C et al. Epidemiology of taeniosis/cysticercosis in Europe, a systematic review: eastern Europe. Parasites & Vectors. 2018;**11**(1):569

[19] Kabululu ML et al. Aggregation of *Taenia solium* cysticerci in pigs: Implications for transmission and control. Parasite Epidemiol Control. 2023;**22**:e00307

[20] Meester M et al. A quantitative risk assessment for human *Taenia solium* exposure from home slaughtered pigs in European countries. Parasites & Vectors. 2019;**12**(1):82

[21] Abuseir S. Meat-borne parasites in the Arab world: A review in a one health perspective. Parasitology Research. 2021;**120**(12):4153-4166

[22] Pinilla M et al. Anti-cysticercus antibodies in pigs and pig breeders in María La Baja, Colombia. Global Journal of Health Science. 2018;**10**:1

[23] Galán-Puchades MT, Fuentes MV. About people, pig movements and pork 'tapeworms'. Veterinary Parasitology. 2015;**214**(1-2):229-230

[24] Shonyela SM et al. An epidemiological survey of porcine cysticercosis in Nyasa District, Ruvuma Region, Tanzania. Parasite Epidemiol Control. 2017;**2**(4):35-41

[25] Donadeu M et al. A hyperendemic focus of porcine cystic echinococcosis in the Banke District of Nepal. Acta Tropica. 2020;**201**:105203

[26] Singh SP et al. Prevalence and distribution of *Taenia solium* cysticercosis in naturally infected pigs in Punjab, India. PLoS Neglected Tropical Diseases. 2018;**12**(11):e0006960

[27] Lightowlers MW, Rolfe R, Gauci CG. *Taenia saginata*: Vaccination against cysticercosis in cattle with recombinant oncosphere antigens. Experimental Parasitology. 1996;**84**(3):330-338

[28] Hewitson JP, Maizels RM. Vaccination against helminth parasite infections. Expert Review of Vaccines. 2014;**13**(4):473-487

[29] Claerebout E, Geldhof P. Helminth vaccines in ruminants: From development to application. The Veterinary Clinics of North America. Food Animal Practice. 2020;**36**(1):159-171

[30] Jazouli M et al. Immunological responses and potency of the EG95NC(−) recombinant sheep vaccine against cystic echinococcosis. Parasitology International. 2020;**78**:102149

[31] Wang YY et al. Optimized codon usage enhances the expression and immunogenicity of DNA vaccine encoding *Taenia solium* oncosphere TSOL18 gene. Molecular Medicine Reports. 2015;**12**(1):281-288

[32] Burgess ST et al. A recombinant subunit vaccine for the control of ovine psoroptic mange (sheep scab). Veterinary Research. 2016;**47**:26

[33] Zhou BY et al. Analysis of immune responses in mice orally immunized with recombinant pMG36e-SP-TSOL18/*Lactococcus lactis* and pMG36e-TSOL18/*Lactococcus lactis* vaccines of *Taenia solium*. Journal of Immunology Research. 2018;**2018**:9262631

Chapter 2

Epidemiology of Taeniosis/Cysticercosis in Humans and Animals

Jasmin Omeragić, Davor Alagić, Sabina Šerić-Haračić and Naida Kapo

Abstract

Taenia saginata, *Taenia solium*, and *Taenia asiatica* popularly known as beef, pork, and Asian tapeworm, are important food-borne parasites. Human taeniosis occurs as a zoonotic consequence of consumption of raw or under-cooked meat contaminated by viable larvae of *T. saginata* (*Cysticercus bovis*), *T. solium* (*Cysticercus cellulosae*) and *T. asiatica* (*Cysticercus viscerotropica*) and further development of their adult forms in human intestines. *T. solium* is highly endemic in pork-consuming poor communities of Asia, Africa, and Latin America, *T. asiatica* is restricted to Asia and is mainly confirmed in South Korea, China, Taiwan, Indonesia, and Thailand, while *T. saginata* is distributed worldwide. Tapeworms cause cysticercosis in pigs and cattle (intermediate hosts) and taeniosis in humans (definitive host). Cysticercosis can also affect people who unintentionally swallow *T. solium* eggs—contaminated soil, water, or food (mainly vegetables) or through self-infection or person-to-person transmission when hygiene practices are insufficient. In humans, human cysticercosis or neurocysticercosis is frequently caused by cysticerci that establish in the central nervous system. Given the effect of *T. solium* on public health and the potential negative effects of *T. saginata* and *T. asiatica* on the economy and trade, defining risk factors, reporting of taeniosis and human cysticercosis is crucial, and surveillance and notification methods in animals should be strengthened.

Keywords: *Taenia solium*, *Taenia saginata*, *Taenia asiatica*, taeniosis, cysticercosis, epidemiology, One Health

1. Introduction

Tapeworms and cysticerci are mentioned during the time of ancient Egypt and Greece. However, their life cycle, including intermediate and definite hosts, are explained in the nineteenth century. Cysticercosis and taeniosis represent food-borne zoonotic infections by the larvae and adult forms of *Taenia saginata* (beef tapeworm), *Taenia solium* (pork tapeworm), and *Taenia asiatica* (Asian tapeworm). These parasites are unique since their life cycle includes humans as definite hosts.

Adult forms of *T. saginata*, *T. solium*, and *T. asiatica* cause human taeniosis. Transmission occurs via consumption of larvae found in animal tissues (beef or pork) and the consequent development of parasites to adult forms in human intestines. Symptoms of intestinal infection are stomachache, intermittent diarrhea, and weight loss, while anal pruritus manifests due to the active migration of proglottids.

Cysticercosis represents infection of tissues by larval stage of Cysticercus (metacestode) found in pigs, cattle, and humans, who in this case can be both intermediate and definite hosts. Larvae of the *T. saginata* are found in the muscles of cattle, larvae of the *T. asiatica* prefer inner organs of pigs (gut and liver), while larvae of the *T. solium* are usually localized in muscles, inner organs, and brain of pigs and humans. After consumption of *T. solium* egg, parasite evolves by larvae (oncospheres) exiting the eggs, which then penetrate the intestine wall and migrate to the eye, striated muscles, and subcutaneous tissue. This is diagnosed as human cysticercosis (HCC). Neurocysticercosis (NCC), occurs when cysticerci migrate to central nervous system tissues and currently it is the most common helminth infection of the nervous system and the leading cause of acquired epilepsy in the world [1]. Hence, *T. solium* is considered as the sole causative agent of NCC in humans with great public health importance, while *T. saginata* and *T. asiatica* are less clinically important. Their main impact is economic losses in animal production. However, the possibility that *T. asiatica* can cause cysticercosis in humans similar as *T. solium* is under investigation due to indications that *T. asiatica* caused several cases of human cysticercosis in Asia [2].

World Health Organization (WHO) considers human cysticercosis and taeniosis as neglected diseases, especially in undeveloped countries where many people live in poor hygiene conditions. Even though taenia-causing infections in humans have a worldwide distribution, cases are mostly reported in regions where cattle and pigs are reared extensively. Therefore, the distribution of each of the three taenia species depends on the culture and nutritional habits (i.e., consummation of raw or undercooked contaminated meat or organs of pigs and cattle) [3–5]. Occurrence of *T. asiatica* is limited to Asia. It is still not reported in Europe, where *T. solium* occurs but not as often, while infections by *T. saginata* are still common. Even though the life cycle of Cestoda is less likely to maintain with appropriate sanitary conditions and good farming practices, infections in such areas still can occur due to migrations. Imported infections increase global distribution into free areas such as the United States of America and Europe. Here infected people contaminate the environment leading to new infections.

Considering the global public health significance of taenia infections, maintaining vigilant surveillance is still needed as a tool to reduce disease incidence as much as possible, as the first step to the eradication of cysticercosis and taeniosis. This chapter summarizes etiology, pathology, and epidemiology of taeniosis/cysticercosis along with science-based approaches to its surveillance as food-borne parasites.

2. Characteristics of the parasites

The genus *Taenia* belongs to the Phylum—Platyhelminthes; Class—Cestoda; Order—Cyclophyllidea; Family—Taeniidae; Genus—*Taenia*. The genus *Taenia* is a highly diverse, paraphyletic group with 45 species identified to date, among which *T. solium*, *T. saginata*, and *T. asiatica* are infectious to humans.

T. asiatica differs from *T. solium* and *T. saginata* by morphological characteristics such as the scolex, mature and gravid proglottids of adults, and the scolex and bladder surface in the larval stage [6]. Today, the characterization of *T. saginata*, *T. solium*, and *T. asiatica* is based on molecular identification and determinations of the mitochondrial genome sequence. The complete mitochondrial genome sequence is available. The difference in the genome between *T. asiatica* and *T. saginata* is 4.6%, while *T. solium* differs by 11% [7]. *T. asiatica* is a relatively recently described species and received much attention in past decades. Discovery came from the paradoxical observation of a high prevalence of taeniosis caused by a *T. saginata*-like tapeworm in humans who did not consume beef, and the consequent description of the complete mitochondrial genome of "new" species. Experimental studies conducted in the 1980s and 1990s clearly demonstrated that the life cycle of *T. asiatica* is comparable to that of *T. saginata*, except that pigs are the preferred intermediate hosts and the liver is the preferred larval site.

Mitochondrial DNA data suggest that *T. saginata* and *T. asiatica* are very closely related [8–10]. *T. saginata* shows high genetic polymorphism (0.2–0.8%), while the genetic diversity of *T. asiatica* appears to be minimal, indicating that this parasite may be on the verge of extinction. However, research has shown the existence of hybrids between *T. asiatica* and *T. saginata*, reviving the issue of *T. asiatica*'s genetic diversity and its position as a distinct species. The identification of *T. saginata* and *T. asiatica* is by morphological and molecular characteristics and observed differences in the life cycle [6]. Genetic variation within the species *T. solium* was until recently almost unknown, even though investigations are ongoing. DNA analysis of *T. solium* isolates from around the world indicate variations between two geographic regions, Asia and Africa/South America, where *T. solium* appears as two genotypes and second is the Asian and the American/African genotype [11]. Analysis of the mitochondrial DNA of *T. saginata* shows great variation indicating greater complexity of this parasite species compared to *T. solium* [12].

2.1 Morphology of the parasites

The three morphological forms of the parasites are adults, eggs, and larvae. Tapeworms of the genus *Taenia* are flat, white or yellowish, and very long-segmented parasites. *T. solium* has a length of 2–8 m, while *T. saginata* and *T. asiatica* are thicker and wider and can be longer. The head or scolex (attachment organ) has four shoots and a rostellum that may contain hooks (*T. solium*), be unhooked and depressed (*T. saginata*), or with rudimentary hooks (*T. asiatica*). Hooks of *T. solium* make a crown with two rows of 22–32 hooks, whose size is 159–173 μm. The scolex is the size of a pinhead, followed by a short and undivided region, the neck. In *T. saginata* the neck is longer and thinner, and in *T. solium* thicker and shorter. The neck continues with a long chain of proglottids or segments (called strobilas). The strobila resembles a ribbon and may consist of several thousand proglottids. Proglottids have different developmental stages: proximal are immature, followed by mature proglottids and distal proglottids containing eggs and gradually increasing in size. The posterior end of the tapeworm has the widest, longest, and oldest proglottids [13–15]. Mature proglottids have both male and female reproductive organs. The female reproductive apparatus includes an ovary, a closed uterus with branches—an ootype, a single mass of bile glands, and a lateral genital pore. Male organs consist of testes (follicles), vas deferens, and cirrus. The uterus in the gravid proglottid of *T. saginata* has 15–30 lateral branches compared to *T. solium* with 7–13 branches. On average, adult *T. solium* has about 1000 proglottids, each containing 50,000 eggs; adult *T. saginata* has about 1000–2000 proglottids, each with 100,000 eggs; while adult *T. asiatica* has 700–900 proglottids, with 80,000 eggs each.

The eggs are spherical, 20–50 μm in size, and morphologically indistinguishable between species of the Taeniidae family. Each egg contains a multicellular embryo with six hooks, hence called a hexanth embryo or oncosphere. Manny eggs released from the definitive host are fully embryonated and infectious. *T. saginata* eggs are infectious to cattle, *T. solium* to both pigs and humans, and *T. asiatica* eggs are infectious to pigs. Because of their resistance to desiccation, eggs can survive for days or months in the environment, in soil, or in water.

Cysticercus *T. solium* (*Cysticercus cellulosae*) is found in the liver, brain, and skeletal muscles of pigs 6 days after infection, while in humans they can be located in the nervous system, eye, heart, muscles, and subcutaneous tissue. A mature cysticercus is usually spherical or oval, white or yellow, 0.5 and 1.5 cm in size, and has a transparent wall, through which the scolex is visible. Cysticerci have two chambers: an inner one containing the scolex and a spiral canal surrounding an outer fluid-containing chamber. The racemous form of cysticercus appears as a large, round, lobulated bladder, limited by a delicate wall or resembles a cluster 10–20 cm in size containing 60 ml of fluid. The most important characteristic of the racemous form is that the scolex cannot be clearly seen. Young cysticerci cause mild inflammation in the surrounding tissue, while mature lead to a stronger immune reaction [16, 17]. Following ingestion by the final host, the pores of the bladder wall expand, resulting in the release of the scolex [18].

Cysticercus *T. saginata* (*Cysticercus bovis*), is a 1 cm wide oval bladder, filled with fluid and containing an invaginated scolex without hooks. Cysticercus are localized in the skeletal muscles of cattle, however, there are sporadic reports of cysticercosis in llamas, pronghorn, oryx, topi and other antelopes, gazelles, wildebeests, and giraffes [19]. These intermediate hosts are infected by grazing.

Cysticercus of *T. asiatica* (*Cysticercus viscerotropica*) is smaller than *T. saginata* with a diameter of approximately 2–3 mm. Both have a scolex with a round rostellum surrounded by four symmetrically placed suckers, while *T. asiatica* has two rows of rudimentary hooks that usually do not develop into morphologically recognizable hooks. Cysticerci of *T. asiatica* are found in domestic and wild pigs and develop in the liver and extrahepatic organs, but not in the muscles [20, 21].

Animals carrying cysticerci are usually asymptomatic while muscle stiffness occurs in extremely severe infections. *C. bovis* and *C. cellulosae* do not develop severe pathology in cattle and pigs unless vital organs, such as the heart, are massively infested.

2.2 The life cycle of the parasites

Parasites of the family Taeniidae uniquely require two obligate hosts (mammalians): a carnivorous/omnivorous definitive host for the adult tapeworm stage and an herbivorous/omnivorous intermediate host for the larval (cysticercus) stage. The life cycle begins when herbivores/omnivores as intermediate hosts ingest plants, food, or water contaminated with taeniid eggs (or gravid proglottids). In the intestines, oncospheres hatch, activate, invade the intestinal wall, and migrate to tissues and organs, where they develop into cysticerci.

When the definitive host carnivore/omnivore eats raw or undercooked pork (*T. solium*, *T. asiatica*) and beef (*T. saginata*) containing fluid-filled cysticerci, the cyst (bladder) gets dissolved and the inverted scolex evacuates under the stimulus of the host's digestive enzymes. The scolex embeds in the intestinal wall, and the neck buds and the strobila is formed. As the adult parasite grows, the release of gravid proglottids begins, and the first shedding occurs between 8 and 12 days after infection. New eggs may appear in the feces of the definitive host within 6–9 weeks, initiating the next cycle of infection [12].

People are infected in three ways:

- by swallowing undercooked/raw beef containing the encysted larval stage (*T. saginata*),
- by swallowing undercooked/raw pork containing the encysted larval stage (*T. solium, T. asiatica*), and
- by ingestion of food (mainly vegetables) or water contaminated with taenia eggs.

3. Epidemiology and public health importance of the parasites

The taeniosis/cysticercosis complex represents a group of zoonoses that are extremely important for public health, and are still endemic in countries of Africa, Asia, and South America (**Table 1**) [22, 23]. In addition to recognition as neglected food-borne zoonotic diseases in many underdeveloped regions, they are also recognized as a significant cause of economic losses in livestock production and pose a danger of spreading in developed countries.

3.1 Epidemiology of *T. solium*

Estimates are that millions of people worldwide are infected with *T. solium*, a tapeworm with more important clinical significance than the other two taenia species. In addition, infections with *T. solium* have greater importance in economically undeveloped countries with poor sanitary conditions, practices of inappropriate cooking and meat processing, extensive pig farming, and low awareness about taeniosis and cysticercosis.

Taeniosis and cysticercosis are endemic in the Andean region of South America, Brazil, Central America, and Mexico; China, the Indian subcontinent, Southeast Asia; and sub-Saharan Africa (**Figure 1**) [25]. In non-endemic countries, that is, many European countries, the USA, Canada, and Australia, reporting of HCC is due to increased consumption of pork, travel, and an increased flow of immigrants [26, 27].

Epidemiological studies estimate 2.56 million human taeniosis cases worldwide and 8.3 cases of cysticercosis [28–31], including at least 400,000 symptomatic cases in South America [32], 1.5–3 million cases in sub-Saharan Africa [29], and 3–7 million cases of HCC in China [32]. Prevalence figures vary in these countries but are usually less than 1:1000 for taeniosis, 1–10% for HCC (undifferentiated cysticercosis and neurocysticercosis), and up to 20–40% for porcine cysticercosis. Estimated seroprevalences are; for *T. solium* in Africa 17.3%, South America 13%, and Asia 15.6% [26]. Children get NCC less often than adults, probably due to a shorter exposure time and/or a different immune response. Likewise, there is no significant differences in the prevalence of HCC between genders or different genetic predispositions in humans.

In most African countries where pigs are raised extensively, cysticercosis caused by *T. solium* is extremely widespread. In the previous decades, this zoonosis in Africa receives more attention due to the recognition of the importance of NCC in

Parasite species	Definitive (intermediate) host	Stages in humans	Stage that infects humans	Human taeniosis/ HCC/NCC	Cysticercosis in animals
T. saginata	Human (Cattle)	Adult tapeworms in intestine	Larvae in undercooked beef	Prevalent in Africa, Southeast Asia, South Asia, and Latin America	Central and East Africa, East, Southeast and South Asia (absent in Japan), and Latin America; low prevalence in Europe
T. solium	Human (pigs, humans)	Adult tapeworms in intestine Cysticercus	Larvae in undercooked pork Eggs in food or water contaminated with human feces	Cosmopolitan, and highly prevalent in Central and South America, Western and Central Africa, Russia, India, Pakistan, China, and Southeast Asia	South America, Asia, Western and Central Africa
T. asiatica	Human (pigs, cattle, goats)	Adult tapeworms in intestine	Larvae in undercooked pork	Prevalent in Taiwan, South Korea, Indonesia, the Philippines, Thailand, China, Vietnam, Japan, and Nepal	East and Southeast Asian countries

Table 1.
Characteristics and distribution of T. saginata, T. solium and T. asiatica.

the etiology of epilepsy. Likewise, data from West and Central Africa suggest that human cysticercosis often does not reflect a true picture of the situation, in contrast to reported prevalences of porcine cysticercosis. Regions of hyperendemicity are in Africa [33] where a high prevalence of cysticercosis in pigs is accompanied by frequent infections with *T. solium* in humans (HCC/NCC). In West Africa, cysticercosis caused by *T. solium* in pigs and humans is reported in Benin, Zambia, Cameroon, Burkina-Faso, Ghana, Côte d'Ivoire, Senegal, and Togo. Although official data are lacking, *T. solium* is probably present in a number of other West African countries [34]. In Central African countries, pig and human cysticercosis are (hyper) endemic in Rwanda, Burundi, the Democratic Republic of Congo, Cameroon, and Chad [34]. Epidemiological studies carried out in Togo and Benin revealed that the prevalence of HCC in Togo was 2.4% and 1.3% in Benin. In some regions of Nigeria, the prevalence of porcine cysticercosis was 20.5%, while the prevalence of taeniosis 8.6%. However, it is surprising that not a single case of HCC/NCC is reported, although epilepsy is very common. Epidemiological data on HCC clearly indicate that, with the exception of predominantly Muslim countries

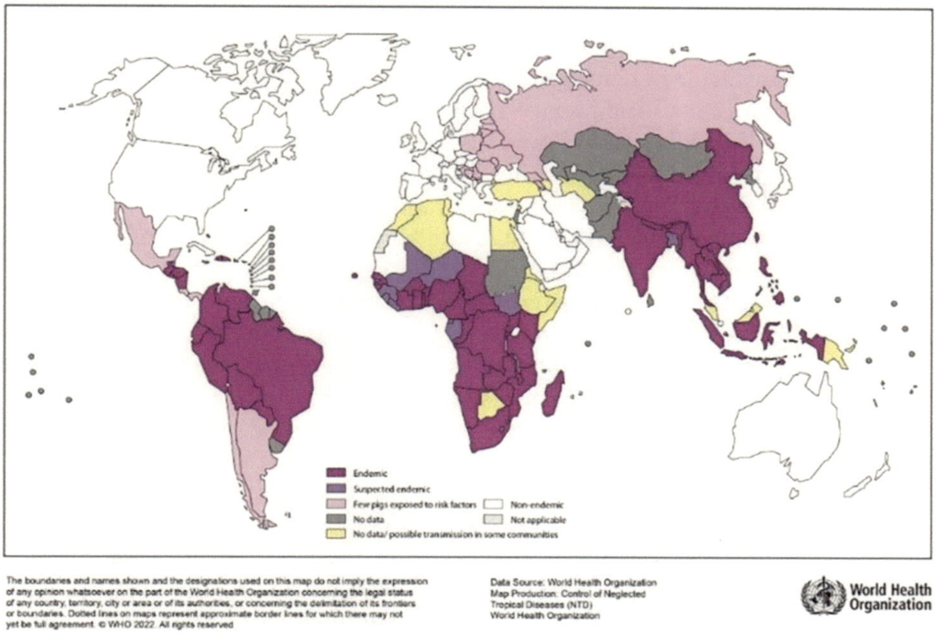

Figure 1.
Worldwide distribution of T. solium infection in 2022 [24].

in North Africa, cysticercosis caused by *T. solium* is endemic in all regions of Africa [35]. Thus, cysticercosis is probably one of the main causes of epilepsy in Cameroon with an incidence rate of as much as 44.6% [36, 37]. Although there is a significant association between cysticercosis and acquired epilepsy in Africa, research on this topic is lacking [35].

In Eastern and Southern African countries, *T. solium* is a serious public health and agricultural problem [38, 39]. Based on available information, annual losses due to cysticercosis in pigs in 10 West and Central African countries amount to around 25 million euros. The financial losses caused by HCC are very difficult to estimate, but they certainly exceeded burden of diseases on the animal side. Because NCC is an important cause of epilepsy, complex treatment dramatically increases the burden of the disease due to the social stigma and discrimination that accompanies the condition. The actual prevalence of cysticercosis caused by *T. solium* in pigs and humans in Central and West Africa is still underestimated due to unreliable data and lack of awareness and diagnostic capacity.

Available data from South America indicate a very significant risk of infection with *T. solium* in humans, although prevalence rates vary from country to country. For example, studies in Honduras, Peru, Mexico, and Guatemala reveal neurological symptoms of NCC in rural populations in 9–18% of residents [40]. Mexico is one of the countries with the highest prevalence of the disease, ranging from 0.2 to 3.4%. NCC in humans in Mexico has often been confirmed post-mortem as the cause of 4–13% of deaths. The reported prevalence of cysticercosis in pigs in Mexico, determined in slaughterhouses, is 0.2%, which is extremely low and does not represent a realistic estimate, as there are a large number of unconfirmed cases [40]. Data on the epidemiology of cysticercosis in most South American countries are unreliable due to a lack of official disease reporting and databases.

Fewer hospitalizations due to cysticercosis were reported in Brazil, Ecuador, and Mexico, as well as reductions in mortality rates in Brazil and in ambulatory cases care in Mexico. Data available in Ecuador compile all forms of cysticercosis, while data on HCC and NCC from Brazil and Mexico allow us to determine that NCC accounts for approximately 90% of all recorded cases of cysticercosis. Thus, the trend of confirmation of cysticercosis in pigs results in higher confirmation of NCC in humans. The trend of NCC burden in Colombia increased significantly between 2009 and 2019 [41]. Serological surveys of HCC and NCC conducted in Colombia from 2008 to 2010 showed high human exposure to *T. solium* [41].

The trend of increasing seropositivity with age is not surprising given that *T. solium* antibodies probably persist for several years. Seropositivity may be an indicator of lifetime prior exposure. In Colombia, *T. solium* antibodies were confirmed more in women than men. This data is consistent with the results of numerous other studies conducted in South America [42–45]. In contrast, in other endemic areas, such as sub-Saharan Africa, males are associated with an increased risk of exposure and higher antibody positivity [46].

Due to human migration, HCC and NCC are also reported in developed countries, such as the USA, where HCC is predominantly an imported disease with a high prevalence in immigrants [47, 48]. In Western Europe, cysticercosis was under control during the last century, but with a significant increase in connection with immigration. Imported human cases are reported from 1990 to the present in all countries except Iceland [49]. Most of the cases are confirmed in Portugal and Spain, but suspected indigenous cases are rare. Simultaneously, cases of cysticercosis in pigs are sporadically reported [50, 51]. In Eastern European countries, the prevalence of cysticercosis exceeds the occurrence in Western Europe. Cases of infection are confirmed in 15 out of 22 countries with the largest number of diagnoses in Romania and Serbia, considered as autochthonous cases [49]. In cases of taeniosis, species identification was not performed [49].

In Asia, taeniosis/cysticercosis has been occurring for several hundred years, but until recently has not received much attention. Consequently, epidemiological data for some areas of the continent do not exist. Data on taeniosis are more available than on cysticercosis [52]. Taeniosis and cysticercosis caused by *T. solium* are common in Bali and Indonesia [53]. In the serological survey in Bali, 21% of people were positive for cysticercosis [54]. Taeniosis is widespread especially among the non-Muslim population, although it is not always certain which species of Taenia is a cause. Cysticercosis is confirmed in India, especially in the north [55]. NCC is confirmed in 50% of patients with epileptic seizures in India. Infections with *T. solium* are reported in Thailand [56], South Korea [57], Taiwan [58], and Nepal [59]. In Nepal, a surprisingly high rate of taeniosis of 50% is found in areas with extensive pig farming. In China, the average prevalence of *T. solium* taeniosis in the investigated regions ranged from 0.05 to 15% [59]. In endemic areas, pig cysticercosis prevalence varied from 0.4 to 15%, and occasionally up to 40%.

3.2 Epidemiology of *T. saginata*

T. saginata has a global distribution; however, the taeniosis it causes is of particular importance in Africa, South America, and Asia [60, 61]. In contrast to *T. solium*, it is considered that *T. saginata* represents a less serious public health problem because this taeniosis rarely leads to serious clinical signs and symptoms in humans. *T. saginata* also leads to significant economic losses, especially in livestock production, and represents a serious problem when it comes to food safety.

Ingestion of *T. saginata* eggs cannot cause cysticercosis in humans, and the public health impact of this parasite is limited to intestinal infection (taeniosis). A risk factor for taeniosis caused by *T. saginata* in humans is the consumption of raw or undercooked beef. According to the prevalence of *T. saginata* an area can fall into one of three categories: (i) highly endemic areas with a prevalence exceeding 10%; (ii) areas with moderate prevalence; and (iii) regions with a prevalence below 0.1% or free of infection. Highly endemic areas include the Central and East African countries (Ethiopia, Kenya, and the Democratic Republic of the Congo) [62]. Endemic areas appear in the Caucasus, Turkey, Iran, Central Asian regions (**Figure 2**), and in the Mediterranean (Syria, Lebanon, and the countries of the former Yugoslavia). The prevalence of taeniosis in humans and cysticercosis in cattle is particularly high in Africa, South America, and some parts of Asia [64].

Research on the prevalence of *T. saginata* in Asia indicates the highest occurrence in the Philippines (33.7%), Pakistan (7%), Vietnam (5.8%), Indonesia (4.6%), Nepal (4.3%), and India (3.8%). In highly endemic regions, for example, Ethiopia, Bali, and Tibet, the prevalence of taeniosis is 22–27%. Cases of taeniosis are reported in Angola, Ethiopia, Kenya, Madagascar, Malawi, South Africa, Tanzania, Uganda, Zambia, and Zimbabwe. In Sichuan and Yunnan provinces of southwestern China, Bali, and Indonesia, raw beef is a delicacy. Consequently, in these rural areas, the prevalence of taeniosis in humans is higher than 20% [65].

T. saginata infections in North America are rare, except in cases where livestock and humans live in close proximity and where poor sanitation prevails. The prevalence of *T. saginata* (under 0.5%) is low in the USA, Canada, Australia, South America, and some countries of the western Pacific, but is slightly higher in Central America [66]. In Europe, infection with *T. saginata* is still endemic in some regions, although the prevalence is low (usually <0.05%) [61].

Taeniosis/cysticercosis caused by *T. saginata* is largely considered a neglected disease in southern and eastern Africa. The reason is low confirmation of infection in cattle, lack of data on the impact of the infection on livestock production

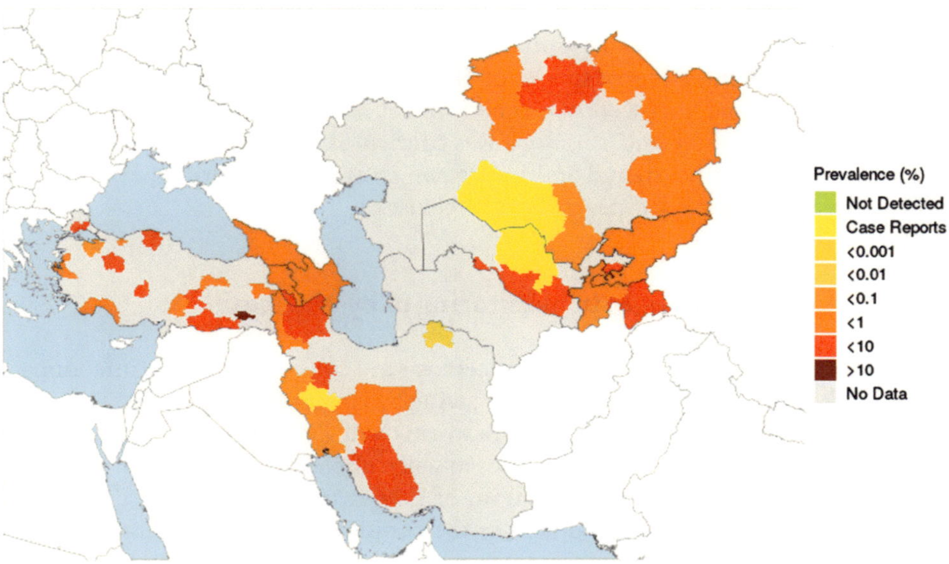

Figure 2.
Prevalence of human taeniosis in central and western Asia and the Caucasus [63].

and economy, and viewing the disease in humans as a minor health problem. Nevertheless, the presence of cysticercosis in cattle is a clear indicator of inadequate sanitary conditions, inadequate meat inspection and human habits that may favor transmission.

The prevalence of cysticercosis in cattle relates to the prevalence of taeniosis in humans. Prevalence in cattle varies from very low (0.03%) in North America and Europe, to very high in Africa and South America (10%–80%) [61, 66]. Cattle cysticercosis in Eastern Europe is generally more frequent than in Western Europe [67]. Information on the prevalence of cysticercosis in cattle in African countries is quite limited, but a very high prevalence of up to 80% is reported (Ethiopia, Botswana, and Nigeria). In Asia, information is also scarce, in general, Japan is considered free of autochthonous bovine cysticercosis based on meat inspection results [68], very high prevalences are reported in various parts of Korea and 2.2% in Indonesia [69]. In contrast, the prevalence is very low in India [70] and the Philippines [71].

3.3 Epidemiology of *T. asiatica*

T. asiatica is overlooked in the context of its impact on the global distribution of taeniosis/cysticercosis in humans. We assume that there are two reasons for the above; the first is the supposedly non-cosmopolitan character of the tapeworm and the second is the close molecular similarity to *T. saginata*, suggesting that *T. asiatica* probably does not cause HCC since *T. saginata* eggs are not infectious to humans. However, *T. saginata* does not cause cysticercosis in pigs, while *T. asiatica* does.

T. asiatica was described in 1993 as a new species of tapeworm that infects humans [6]. Previously, its occurrence in rural communities in Southeast Asia was attributed to *T. saginata* which is morphologically very similar but described in patients who ate raw pork liver but not beef [72]. Currently, there is no specific immunodiagnostic method to confirm *T. asiatica*, and molecular techniques (the only tool for distinguishing between the 3 Taenia species) are not used in routine diagnostics. Hence, the geographic distribution of *T. asiatica* and its ability to cause HCC remain open questions. *T. asiatica* is confirmed in Asia (Korea, China, Japan, Taiwan, Indonesia, Thailand, Nepal, Vietnam, the Philippines, Cambodia, and Myanmar) [72]. In a study conducted in Thailand, all three species of Taenia appeared in communities where undercooked pork and beef were consumed, and at least one dual infection with adult tapeworms *T. solium* and *T. asiatica* was confirmed by DNA analysis. In many countries of East, Southeast, and South Asia, which are rich in cultural, ethnic, and religious diversity, all three types of Taenia coexist.

4. Meat inspection changes in monitoring of cysticercosis

Bovine cysticercosis and porcine cysticercosis are common parasitic infections of mainly skeletal muscles of bovines and swine by larval stages (cysticerci) of the two large tapeworms *T. saginata* (beef tapeworm) and *T. solium* (pork tapeworm). Human taeniosis occurs as a zoonotic consequence of consumption of raw or undercooked meat contaminated by viable larvae of *T. saginata* (*C. bovis*) and *T. solium* (*C. cellulosae*) and further development of their adult forms in human intestines. *T. asiatica* was also described as the new taenia species that parasitize in humans as definitive hosts [6], which geographical distribution is limited to Asia [72]. In addition, unlike *T. saginata* and *T. solium,* this tapeworm infects pigs, cattle, goats, and certain monkey species as intermediate hosts, in which cysticerci are predominantly located in liver [73]. *T. asiatica* is not considered to cause human cysticercosis [74]. Other *Taenia* spp., such as *T. multiceps,* that parasitize in domestic and wild animals, do not normally invade humans, although cases of coenurosis (infection of the brain, spinal cord, and eyes with *Coenurus cerebralis* as the larval stage of *T. multiceps*) have been reported in humans [75, 76]. Human cysticercosis or neurocysticercosis is another zoonotic form of food-borne infection by *T. solium*, which occurs as a life-threatening illness subsequently to invasion of the central nervous system by *C. cellulosae*. Human cysticercosis is considered as the most dominant helminthic infection of the nervous system and a major global cause of acquired epilepsy [77, 78]. The diseases caused by *T. saginata* and *T. solium* are worldwide reported, with estimates on their occurrence ranging regionally, as well from country to country. As for Bosnia and Herzegovina, the available data are scarce and limited, but cases of human and bovine cysticercosis were reported [79].

Due to the zoonotic potential, bovine, porcine and other forms of animal cysticercosis are notifiable to the World Organization for Animal Health [80]. As for the European Union (EU), monitoring of cysticercosis in the EU Member States (MS) becomes compulsory depending on the epidemiological situation, as regulated by List B of Annex I of the Directive 2003/99/EC [81]. Based on the monitoring data, each MS must evaluate the trends and sources of zoonoses, zoonotic agents, and antimicrobial resistance in their territory and send annual national reports to the European Commission. Each year the national reports from all MS are evaluated and published by European Food Safety Authority (EFSA) as the EU Summary Report on the trends and sources of zoonoses, zoonotic agents, and antimicrobial resistance in the EU. Since 2019, the annual EU Summary Reports on zoonoses, zoonotic agents and foodborne outbreaks have been renamed the "EU One Health Zoonoses Summary Report" (EUOHZ), which is co-authored by EFSA and European Centre for Disease Prevention and Control. The latest published EUOHZ report for 2021 [82] included very scarce data on *Cysticercus* spp. in several animal host species from only eight MS. Frequency of cysticerci detected in bovine carcasses at slaughterhouses was 0.271% (74 positive out of the 27,326 inspected) in Luxembourg, 0.111% in Belgium (857 positive out of the 770,235 inspected), 0.009% in Slovakia (3 positive out of 34,771) and Slovenia (11 positive out of 123,961), 0.005% in Spain (125 out of 2,332,666), while Sweden reported only one positive out of 411,650 inspected cattle carcasses. As for inspected pork, cysticerci were found in 0.001% (7 positive out of 675,234 checked) and in 0.007% (2902 positive out of 41,059,466 inspected) pig carcasses in Slovakia and Spain, respectively. Spain also detected cysticerci in 33 of 111,100 wild boars (0.03%), 17,332 out of 799,767 goats (2.18%), 200,810 out of 7,077,050 sheep (2.84%), and in 110 out of 4544 inspected solipeds (2.42%). Moreover, cysticerci were not detected in 2,200,672 cattle, pig and wild boar carcasses inspected in Finland, in 65,334 cattle, pig, sheep or goat carcasses collected in Malta, or in 7415 mouflons and 118,899 deer inspected in Spain [82].

The existing problem of low reporting data on cysticercosis in EU has been previously recognized and evaluated by the EFSA Panel on Biological Hazard [83] and other scientific report submitted to EFSA [84], where it has been generally assumed that cysticercosis is more frequent in animal and human populations in the EU, with very low sensitivity of slaughterhouse inspection recognized as the main reason for underreporting of cysticercosis.

The major constraint with regard to monitoring of cysticercosis is the lack of a "gold-standard" reference diagnostic test that would solely ensure a high level of confidence in detecting the disease, particularly in animals with low parasite burdens [85]. Monitoring of cysticercosis is performed by post-mortem meat inspection at the slaughterhouse. Meat inspection by visual inspection, palpation and incision of appropriate organs was originally introduced at the end of nineteenth century by Robert Ostertag [86, 87]. In Bosnia and Herzegovina, post-mortem meat inspection is currently imposed by specific national regulation [88], which is completely harmonized with Regulation (EC) No 854/2004 [89], imposing mandatory visual inspection of all surfaces of each carcass of slaughtered animals by the official veterinarian. In addition, the official veterinarian may require carcasses of bovine animals over 6 months old, and domestic swine over 4 weeks old to be submitted for post-mortem inspection split lengthways into half carcasses down the spinal column. Furthermore, if the inspection so necessitates, the official veterinarian may also require any head or any carcass to be split lengthwise. Also, specific examinations such as palpation and incision of parts of the carcasses (such as predilection locations for cysticerci; tongue, esophagus, diaphragm, internal and external masseters, pericardium and heart), offal and laboratory tests, must be carried out to, among other reasons, detect the presence of a zoonotic disease such as cysticercosis. Also, requirements for systematic visual inspection, palpation, and incisions of carcasses from bovines under and above 6 weeks old, and for domestic swine carcasses are specified as well. In addition to the specified post-mortem meat inspection procedures as the minimum requirements for the examination for cysticercosis in bovine animals over 6 weeks old and swine, the use of specific serological tests is also allowed. In the case of bovines over 6 weeks old, incision of the masseters at post-mortem inspection is not compulsory when a specific serological test is used, as well as when bovine animals over 6 weeks old have been raised on a holding officially certified to be free of cysticercosis. Finally, it is stated that carcasses infected with cysticerci must be declared as unfit for human consumption and condemned. However, when the animal is not generally infected with cysticerci, the uninfected parts may be declared as fit for human consumption after having undergone a cold treatment [90], such as kept at temperatures below –10°C minimally for 2 weeks or at –7°C for at least 3 weeks [91].

Diagnostic sensitivity of the post-mortem visual inspection lower than 30% (or reduced to 1% for very low parasite burden and localized infections) and its questionable specificity triggered by possible misdiagnosis are known, which results in low official reporting and underestimated prevalence of cysticercosis [92]. Also, the effectiveness of visual inspection, incision and palpation in detecting cysticercosis-positive carcasses greatly rely on the level of training, experience, and skills of official veterinarians, which makes the post-mortem meat inspection very subjective, time-demanding, and laborious and results in absence of proficiency scheme, ring trials and standardization of the method [86, 92], and in the lack of a proficiency scheme or ring trials. In addition to evident financial costs and losses due to cysticercosis and taeniosis [92], these are the main reasons that alternative diagnostic techniques have been studied to be introduced in meat inspection procedures and improve diagnostics of cysticercosis.

Mostly deficient and unspecific clinical manifestation of the disease in bovines and swine reflects in overall ineffectiveness to screen cysticercosis in animals during the ante-mortem inspection. Bovine cysticercosis does not cause clinically apparent symptoms in infected animals, except for ones with observed multi-organ infestation with *C. bovis*. Gholami et al. [93] described obvious symptoms, such as different degrees of lethargy, dullness, unthriftiness, and reluctance to move in feedlot cattle in Iran, in which post-mortem inspection showed multi-organ infection with the cysticerci, such as heart, tongue muscle, masticatory muscle, lungs, and liver. The authors reported that the most and least invaded organs were heart (100%) and liver (14.28%), respectively. On the other hand, clinical manifestation of porcine cysticercosis largely depends on localization of *C. cellulosae* in infected pigs, which is primarily in muscle tissue and the brain [94]. Predilection of the cysticerci for the brain of infected pigs may trigger disorders of the central nervous system as dominant clinical manifestations of porcine neurocysticercosis. Trevisan et al. [95] reported that clinical signs of porcine neurocysticercosis included severe seizures with stereotyping walking in circles, chewing motions, foamy salivation, and ear stiffening, accompanied with tonic muscle contractions followed by a generalized rapid loss of muscular function and collapse of the animal. Even though the authors reported a significant positive association between seizures and age of the animals ($p < 0.001$), they observed the seizures in only two of 16 infected animals, while significant relations between seizures and total number, distribution and localization of cysticerci in the brain were not reported. In addition to seizures, less severe signs of porcine cysticercosis may include excessive salivation, excessive blinking and tearing, and presence of subconjunctival nodule [96], as well as dullness, sluggishness, somnolence, apathy, and loss of consciousness [97, 98].

Unlike irregular and non-pathognomonic neurological manifestations of porcine cysticercosis, localization of *C. cellulosae* in tongue muscular tissue was the rationale for antemortem lingual palpation (tongue inspection) as a rapid and inexpensive tool for pig producers, buyers, and veterinarians to screen cysticercosis in pigs [98]. Dorny et al. [99] reported that lingual palpation was 100% specific in detecting cysticercotic pigs if performed correctly by experienced persons and combined by the visual inspection of the tongue base. However, the authors estimated the overall sensitivity of tongue inspection at only 21%, which confirmed previous observations that the sensitivity of detecting cysticercosis-positive pigs solely by lingual inspection is greatly limited if the tongue is not heavily invaded with the cysts [100]. The sensitivity of tongue inspection fluctuates depending on the infection intensity and the test is suitable only in the areas where porcine cysticercosis is highly endemic [101].

Serological techniques, such as ELISA, have been widely employed to screen cysticercosis in pigs [101–103] and in bovines [104–106], where the estimated values for sensitivity and specificity of the applied tests varied greatly. Chembensofu et al. [103] evaluated the performance of circulating antigen detection (Ag-ELISA) against full carcass dissection as the gold standard method in detecting naturally *T. solium*-infected pigs in Zambia. The authors reported the Ag-ELISA specificity and sensitivity in detecting infected carcasses to be 67% and 68%, respectively, and increasing to 90 and 100% for the detection of carcasses with one or more viable cysticerci, and more than 10 viable cysts, respectively. Using a similar approach, Kabulu et al. [101] estimated Ag-ELISA sensitivity and specificity in detecting *T. solium* cysticerci in naturally infected pigs in Tanzania to be 82.7% and 86.3%, respectively, and concluded that the Ag-ELISA test used in the study is more reliable in ruling out *T. solium* cysticercosis in pigs, than in confirming it, since the positive and negative predictive values of the test were 35.2% and 98.2%, respectively. Using an Ag-ELISA test to estimate the prevalence of bovine cysticercosis, Dorny et al. [104] examined 1164 serum samples of cattle slaughtered in Belgium and detected 3.09% cysticercosis-positive serum samples, while the routine post-mortem meat inspection of the same cattle detected the disease only in 0.26% carcasses, which underlines very low sensitivity as the most important disadvantage of the routine meat inspection in detecting cysticercosis. Eichenberger et al. [106] assessed diagnostic values of various ELISA tests and the EU mandatory antemortem visual meat inspection for detecting *T. saginata* cysticercosis in 793 dairy cows slaughtered in three EU-approved slaughterhouses in Switzerland. In the absence of the "gold-standard" reference diagnostic test, the results of the mandatory meat inspection test and four ELISA tests were further analyzed by use of Bayesian inference. The reported Bayesian estimates of the ELISA tests sensitivity ranged from 14.3% (95% CI: 8.7–21.5) for monoclonal Ab-ELISA to 81.6% (95% CI: 70.1–92.0) for *T. saginata* metacestode excretory/secretory antigen ELISA, while the reported specificity values were between 84.7% (95% CI: 81.6–87.6) for commercial synthesized purified peptide ELISA and 96.3% (95% CI: 93.5–99.0) for *T. saginata* metacestode excretory/secretory antigen ELISA. Sensitivity of the EU routine visual meat inspection was very low, estimated at 15.6% (95% CI: 10.0–23.3), with assumed specificity of 100 [106].

Obviously, the low sensitivity and specificity of the EU mandatory routine visual meat inspection in detecting cysticercosis at slaughterhouses by can be enhanced by combining it with ELISA testing. However, some properties of the ELISA techniques, such as lack of officially registered and commercially available tests for bovine cysticercosis [84] and requirement to be performed by a specialized laboratory [92], make serological techniques unsuitable for routine use to detect cysticercosis in cattle and pigs. In addition, introduction of serological tests for monitoring cysticercosis in animals would greatly increase overall costs related to the disease monitoring. As projected by Jansen et al. [92], employment of an Ag-ELISA test (with estimated sensitivity of 36.37% and specificity of 99.36%) at cattle slaughter would greatly reduce the estimated prevalence of bovine cysticercosis in Belgium from 42.5 to 0.6%. However, such an improvement would generate economic losses for the cattle owners up to 21 million EUR and 10 million EUR for the slaughterhouses just in the first year after implementing the Ag-ELISA, which are enormous increases in financial damages if compared to estimated annual loss of 3.5 million EUR and 200,000 EUR without the test, respectively. Other analytical methods used to for the monitoring and reporting *Cysticercus* in animals and foodstuffs in the EU, such as the parasite taxonomic identification, histopathology, and molecular (DNA) methods were found to be deficient in estimates of their sensitivity and/or specificity, and characterized with lower diagnostic throughput and higher estimated costs when compared to the routine meat inspection and ELISA methods and require specialized diagnostic facilities [84], which has not resulted in routine use of serological methods as an alternative to visual meat inspection [91].

Evidently, meat inspection based on the post-mortem visual inspection, palpation, and incision of carcasses with proven low sensitivity and substantial financial burden need to be advanced toward the risk-based meat safety assurance system in order to provide a better public health protection from meat-borne diseases, as suggested by EFSA [107–109]. To enable MS to perform risk analysis essential for risk categorization of animals and an effective implementation of risk-based meat inspection, EFSA proposed Harmonized Epidemiological Indicators (HEIs) for all meat-producing animal species, including pigs [110] and bovines [111]. The proposed HEIs include, among others, prevalence of hazards in animals or meat at different stages of the food production chain, and other criteria, such as animal hygiene indicators or visible carcass contamination. To be measurable against objective criteria and to achieve an acceptable level, each HEI is defined in terms of respective food production stage, analytical/diagnostic method, and required specimens, if applicable. Such an effort and contribution of EFSA resulted in adoption of the current EU meat inspection legislation [112–115]. The main drive for the change in EU legislation has been to boost quality improvement and better use of data collected along the integrated food production chain (Food Chain Information—FCI), which are of pivotal importance for establishing reliable HEIs and consequent risk analysis and risk categorization of animal herds. This should enable the shift from the traditional meat inspection approach to the current risk-based meat safety assurance system in which meat of low risk-animals is visual-only inspected (VOI), while meat of high-risk animals is subject to palpation and/or incision [116]. The VOI approach was initiated by the Regulation (EC) No 854/2004 [89] for indoor-raised finisher pigs, while the current Regulation (EU) No 218/2014 [112] allows VOI for all low-risk pigs. As for bovine carcasses, VOI is legalized by the EU Regulation No 2019/627 [115], since the regulation recognizes the actual risks of cysticerci in various cattle categories, which should enable reduction of manual inspection of the carcasses. However, as recognized by Blagojevic et al. [117], a full benefit from legal introduction of VOI approach has not yet been fully achieved, since reduced incisions cause a further decrease in already low sensitivity of traditional meat inspection in detecting bovine cysticercosis, and the additional costs of alternative serological testing hinder its utilization. Challenges and opportunities in the implementation of the new risk-based meat inspection system were recently studied by Antunovic et al. [116]. The authors identified existing trade agreements with third countries, costs of implementation, and inadequate FCI and resistance from meat inspectors as the most frequent obstacles to implementing the new meat inspection systems. In addition, the stakeholders are more confident in the new systems than in the traditional system, while reduced or equal inspection workload compared to the traditional system was observed.

Therefore, further research and expand of means of employing FCI and HEIs are crucial to reach better risk categorization of and enhanced implementation of risk-based meat safety assurance system which should consequently reduce the workload of veterinary inspection, decrease the related costs for the whole meat industry, improve sensitivity of detecting meat-borne hazards and enhance overall public health protection.

5. Conclusion

The high prevalence of taeniosis and cysticercosis is a reflection of poor sanitary conditions, which are below standards and poor food safety measures. Therefore, in endemic areas there is a need to improve local surveillance, sanitary conditions, diagnostics and the regulatory system.

Author details

Jasmin Omeragić, Davor Alagić, Sabina Šerić-Haračić and Naida Kapo*
Veterinary Faculty, University of Sarajevo, Bosnia and Herzegovina

*Address all correspondence to: naida.kapo@vfs.unsa.ba

IntechOpen

© 2023 The Author(s). Licensee IntechOpen. This chapter is distributed under the terms of the Creative Commons Attribution License (http://creativecommons.org/licenses/by/3.0), which permits unrestricted use, distribution, and reproduction in any medium, provided the original work is properly cited.

References

[1] Bruno E, Bartoloni A, Zammarchi L, et al. Epilepsy and neurocysticercosis in Latin America: A systematic review and meta-analysis. PLoS Neglected Tropical Diseases. 2013;**7**(10):e2480. DOI: 10.1371/journal.pntd.0002480

[2] Gala'n-Puchades MT, Fuentes MV. Human cysticercosis and larval tropism of *Taenia saginata asiatica*. Parasitology Today. 2000;**16**:174. DOI: 10.3347/kjp.2000.38.1.1

[3] Ito A, Budke CM. Culinary delights and travel? A review of zoonotic cestodiases and metacestodiases. Travel Medicine and Infectious Disease. 2014;**12**:582-591. DOI: 10.1016/j.tmaid.2014.06.009

[4] Ito A, Wandra T, Li T, Dekumyoy P, Nkouawa A, Okamoto M, et al. The present situation of human taeniases and cysticercosis in Asia. Recent Patents on Anti-Infective Drug Discovery. 2014;**9**(3):173-185. DOI: 10.2174/1574891x10666150410125711

[5] Sato MO, Nunes CM, Sato M, Waikagul J. *Taenia*. In: Xiao L, Ryan U, Feng Y, editors. Biology of Foodborne Parasites. United States: CRC Press; 2015. pp. 463-480. DOI: 10.1201/b18317

[6] Eom KS, Rim HJ. Morphologic descriptions of *Taenia asiatica* sp. n. The Korean Journal of Parasitology. 1993;**31**(1):1-6. DOI: 10.3347/kjp.1993.31.1.1

[7] Jeon HK, Kim KH, Eom KS. Complete sequence of the mitochondrial genome of *Taenia saginata*: Comparison with *T. solium* and *T. asiatica*. Parasitology International. 2007;**56**:243-246. DOI: 10.1016/j.parint.2007.04.001

[8] Zarlenga DS, McManus DP, Fan PC, Cross JH. Characterization and detection of a newly described Asian Taeniid using cloned Ribosomal DNA fragment and sequence amplification by polymerase chain reaction. Experimental Parasitology. 1991;**72**:174-183

[9] Hoberg EP, Jones A, Rausch RL, Eom KS, Gardner SL. A phylogenetic hypothesis for species of the genus Taenia (Eucestoda: Taeniidae). The Journal of Parasitology. 2000;**86**:89-98. DOI: 10.1645/0022-3395(2000)086[0089

[10] Jeon HK, Eom KS. *Taenia asiatica* and *Taenia saginata*: Genetic divergence estimated from their mitochondrial genomes. Experimental Parasitology. 2006;**113**:58-61. DOI: 10.1016/j.exppara.2005.11.018

[11] Nakao M, Okamoto M, Sako Y, Yamasaki H, Nakaya K, Ito A. A phylogenetic hypothesis for the distribution of two genotypes of the pig tapeworm *Taenia solium* worldwide. Parasitology. 2002;**124**:657-662

[12] Myadagsuren N et al. Taeniasis in Mongolia, 2002-2006. The American Journal of Tropical Medicine and Hygiene. 2007;**77**:342-346

[13] Flisser A. Larval Cestodes. In: Richardson DJ, Krause Pj, editors. Topley & Wilson's Microbiology and Microbial Infections. 9th ed. Arnold: London; 1998. pp. 539-560

[14] Flisser A. Taeniasis and cysticercosis due to Taenia solium. In: Sun T, editor. Progress in Clinical Parasitology. Boca Raton, Fla: CRC; 1994. pp. 77-116

[15] Fan PC, Lin CY, Chen CC, Chung WC. Morphological description of

Taenia saginata asiatica (Cyclophyllidea: Taeniidae) from man in Asia. Journal of Helminthology. 1995;**69**:299-303

[16] Flisser A et al. Praziquantel treatment of porcine brain and muscle *Taenia solium* cisticercosis. 1. Radiological, physiological and histopathological studies. Parasitology Research. 1990;**76**:263-269

[17] Aluja AS, Vargas G. The histopathology of porcine cysticercosis. Veterinary Parasitology. 1988;**28**:65-77

[18] Rabiela MT et al. Evagination of *Taenia solium cysticerci*: A histologic and electron microscopy study. Archives of Medical Research. 2000;**31**:605-607

[19] Nelson GS et al. The significance of wild animals in the transmission of cestodes of medical importance in Kenya. Transactions of the Royal Society of Tropical Medicine and Hygiene. 1965;**59**:507-524

[20] Pawlowski Z, Schultz MG. Taeniasis and cysticercosis (*Taenia saginata*). Advances in Parasitology. 1972;**10**:269-343

[21] Fan PC. The history of *Taeniasis saginata* in Taiwan before world war II. Yonsei Reports in Tropical Medicine. 1995;**26**:13-17

[22] Ito A, Yanagida T, Nakao M. Recent advances and perspectives in molecular epidemiology of *Taenia solium* cysticercosis. Infection, Genetics and Evolution. 2016;**40**:357-367. DOI: 10.1016/j.meegid.2015.06.022

[23] Fabiani S, Bruschi F. Neurocysticercosis in Europe: Still a public health concern not only for imported cases. Acta Tropica. 2013;**128**:18-26. DOI: 10.1016/j.actatropica.2013.06.020

[24] Donadeu M, Bote K, Gasimov E, Kim SH, et al. *Taenia solium*: WHO endemicity map update. Weekly Epidemiological Record. 2022;**17**(97):169-172

[25] Gemmell M, Matyas Z, Pawlowski Z, Soulsby EJL, Larralde C, et al. In: Gemmell M, editor. Guidelines for Surveillance, Prevention and Control of Taeniasis/Cysticercosis. Edinburgh, Scotland: World Health Organization; 1983

[26] Coral-Almeida M, Gabriël S, Abatih EN, Praet N, Benitez W, Dorny P. *Taenia solium* human cysticercosis: A systematic review of sero-epidemiological data from endemic zones around the world. PLoS Neglected Tropical Diseases. 2015;**9**(7):e0003919. DOI: 10.1371/journal.pntd.0003919

[27] Bobes RJ, Fragoso G, Fleury A, et al. Evolution, molecular epidemiology and perspectives on the research of taeniid parasites with special emphasis on *Taenia solium*. Infection, Genetics and Evolution. 2014;**23**:150-160. DOI: 10.1016/j.meegid.2014.02.005

[28] Richards FO Jr. *Cestode zoonoses*: Echinococcosis and Cysticercosis: An emergent and global problem. Emerging Infectious Diseases. 2002;**8**(11):1362. DOI: 10.3201/eid0811.020422

[29] Wandra T, Swastika K, Dharmawan NS, Purba IE, Sudarmaja IM, Yoshida T, et al. The present situation and towards the prevention and control of neurocysticercosis on the tropical island, Bali, Indonesia. Parasites & Vectors. 2015;7(8):148. DOI: 10.1186/s13071-015-0755-z

[30] Craig PS et al. Detection, screening and community epidemiology of taeniid *Cestode zoonoses*: Cystic echinococcosis, alveolar echinococcosis and neurocysticercosis. Advances in Parasitology. 1996;**38**:169-250

[31] Pal Deb K, Carpio A, Sander JWAS. Neurocysticercosis and epilepsy in developing countries. Journal of Neurology, Neurosurgery, and Psychiatry. 2000;**68**(2):137-143

[32] Hendrickx E, Thomas LF, Dorny P, et al. Epidemiology of *Taenia saginata* taeniosis/cysticercosis: A systematic review of the distribution in West and Central Africa. Parasites & Vectors. 2019;**12**:324. DOI: 10.1186/s13071-019-3584-7

[33] Zoli A, SheyNjila O, Assana E, Nguekam JP, Dorny P, Brandt J, et al. Regional status, epidemiology and impact of *Taenia solium* cysticercosis in Western and Central Africa. Acta Tropica. 2003;**87**(1):35-42. DOI: 10.1016/s0001-706x(03)00053-6

[34] Foyaca-Sibat H et al. Accuracy of serological testing for the diagnosis of prevalent neurocysticercosis in outpatients with epilepsy, Eastern Cape Province, South Africa. PLoS Neglected Tropical Diseases. 2009;**3**(12):e562

[35] Velasco Suarez M, Bravo Becherelle MA, Quirasco F. Human cysticercosis: Medical social implications and economic impact. In: Flisser A, Willms K, Laclette JP, Larralde C, Ridaura C, Beltran F, editors. Cysticercosis: Present State of Knowledge and Perspectives. New York: Academic Press; 1982. pp. 47-51

[36] Nkouawa A, Sako Y, Itoh S, Kouojip Mabou A, et al. Serological studies of neurologic helminthic infections in rural areas of Southwest Cameroon: Toxocariasis, cysticercosis and paragonimiasis. PLoS Neglected Tropical Diseases. 2010;**4**:e732. DOI: 10.1371/journal.pntd.0000732

[37] Quet F, Guerchet M, Pion SDS, Ngoungou EB, Nicoletti A, Preux PM. Meta-analysis of the association between cysticercosis and epilepsy in Africa. Epilepsia. 2010;**51**:830-837. DOI: 10.1111/j.1528-1167.2009.02401

[38] Krecek RC, Michael LM, Schantz PM, Ntanjana L, Smith MF, Dorny P, et al. Prevalence of *Taenia solium* cysticercosis in swine from a community-based study in 21 villages of the Eastern Cape province. South African Veterinary Parasitology. 2008;**154**:38-47. DOI: 10.1016/j.vetpar.2008.03.005

[39] Assana E, Lightowlers MW, Zoli AP, Geerts S. *Taenia solium* taeniosis/cysticercosis in Africa: Risk factors, epidemiology and prospects for control using vaccination. Veterinary Parasitology. 2013;**195**(1-2):14-23. DOI: 10.1016/j.vetpar.2012.12.022

[40] Galipó E, Dixon MA, Fronterrè C, et al. Spatial distribution and risk factors for human cysticercosis in Colombia. Parasites & Vectors. 2021;**14**:590. DOI: 10.1186/s13071-021-05092-8

[41] Allan JC, Velasquez-Tohom M, Garcia-Noval J, Torres-Alvarez R, Yurrita P, Fletes C, et al. Epidemiology of intestinal taeniasis in four, rural Guatemalan communities. Tropical Medicine and Parasitology. 1996;**90**(2):157-165

[42] Garcia-Noval J, Allan JC, Fletes C, Moreno E, De Mata F, Torres-Alvarez R, et al. Epidemiology of *Taenia solium* taeniasis and cysticercosis in two rural Guatemalan communities. The American Journal of Tropical Medicine and Hygiene. 1996;**55**(3):282-289

[43] Garcia HH, Araoz R, Gilman RH, Valdez J, Gonzalez AE, Gavidia C, et al. Increased prevalence of cysticercosis and taeniasis among professional fried pork vendors and the general population of a village in the Peruvian highlands. The

American Journal of Tropical Medicine and Hygiene. 1998;**59**(6):902-905

[44] Agudelo-Flórez P, Restrepo BN, Palacio LG. Knowledge and practices concerning taeniasis-cysticercosis in Colombian pig-breeders. Revista de Salud Pública. 2009;**11**(2):191-199. DOI: 10.1590/s0124-00642009000200004 (in Spanish)

[45] Nithiuthai S, Anantaphruti MT, Waikagul J, Gajadhar A. Waterborne zoonotic helminthiases. Veterinary Parasitology. 2004;**126**(1-2):167-193

[46] Serpa JA, White AC Jr. Neurocysticercosis in the United States. Pathogens and Global Health. 2012;**106**(5):256-260. DOI: 10.1179/2047773212Y.0000000028

[47] Carabin H et al. Methods for assessing the burden of parasitic zoonoses: Echinococcosis and cysticercosis. Trends in Parasitology. 2005;**21**:327-333. DOI: 10.1016/j.pt.2005.05.009

[48] Mahajan RC. Geographical distribution of human cysticercosis. In: Flisser A, Willms K, Laclette JP, et al. Cysticercosis: Present State of Knowledge and Perspectives. New York: Academic Press; 1982. pp. 39-46

[49] Laranjo-González M, Devleesschauwer B, Trevisan C, Allepuz A, Sotiraki S, Abraham A, et al. Epidemiology of taeniosis/cysticercosis in Europe, a systematic review: Western Europe. Parasites & Vectors. 2017;**10**(1):349. DOI: 10.1186/s13071-017-2280-8

[50] Herrador Z, Pérez-Molina JA, Henríquez Camacho CA, Rodriguez-Guardado A, Bosch-Nicolau P, Calabuig E, et al. Imported cysticercosis in Spain: A retrospective case series from the +REDIVI Collaborative Network. Travel Medicine and Infectious Disease. 2020;**37**:101683. DOI: 10.1016/j.tmaid.2020.101683

[51] Dorny P, Somoes R, Dang TCT, Nguyen VK, Vereruysse J. Cysticercosis in Cambodia, Laos and Vietnam. The Southeast Asian Journal of Tropical Medicine and Public Health. 2004;**35**:223-226

[52] Rajshekhar V, Durga D, Joshi DD, Doanh NQ, van De N, Xiaonony Z. *Taenia solium* taeniosis/cysticercosis in Asia: Epidemiology, impact and issues. Acta Tropica. 2003;**87**:53-60. DOI: 10.1016/s0001-706x(03)00055-x

[53] Coker Vann MR, Subianto DB, Brown P, Diwan AR, Desowitz R, Garruto RM, et al. ELISA antibodies to cysticerci of *Taenia solium* in human populations. Southeast Asian Journal of Tropical Medicine and Public Health. 1981;**12**(4):499-505

[54] Rajshekhar V. Epidemiology of *Taenia solium* in India and Nepal. The Southeast Asian Journal of Tropical Medicine and Hygiene. 2004;**35**:247-251

[55] Khamboonraung C. On emerging problems in food-borne parasitic zoonoses: Impact on agriculture and public health. The Southeast Asian Journal of Tropical Medicine and Public Health. 1991;**22**:1-7

[56] Eom Keeseon S, Jeon H-K, Rim H-J. Geographical distribution of *Taenia asiatica* and related species. The Korean Journal of Parasitology. 2009;**47**(Suppl):S115

[57] Chen Y, Xu L, Zhou X. Distribution and burden of cysticercosis in China. The Southeast Asian Journal of Tropical Medicine and Public Health. 2004;**35**:231-239. DOI: 10.1016/j.actatropica.2016.01.013

[58] Close PJ, Hotez BP. "Manifesto" for advancing the control and elimination of neglected tropical diseases. PLoS Neglected Tropical Diseases. 2010;**4**:e718. DOI: 10.1371/annotation/53d95072-6329-412d-a5e4-c1a00acd1934

[59] Penfold WJ, Penfold HB, Phillips M. Acquired active immunity in the ox to *Cysticercus bovis*. The Medical Journal of Australia. 1936;**1**:417-423

[60] Pawlowski ZS. *Taenia solium*: Basic biology and transmission. In: Singh G, Prabhakar S, editors. *Taenia solium* Cysticercosis: From Basic to Clinical Sciences. Wallingford, Oxfordshire, UK: CABI Publishing; 2002. pp. 1-14

[61] Petrovic Z, Radovic M, Lavsevic B. Significance and problems of taeniasis in some parts of Yugoslavia. Acta Veterinaria (Yugoslavia). 1982;**32**:31-36

[62] Murrell KD. Epidemiology of taeniosis and cysticercosis. In: Murrell KD, editor. WHO/FAO/OIE Guidelines for the Surveillance, Prevention and Control of Taeniosis/Cysticercosis. Paris: Office International des Epizooties (OIE); 2005. pp. 27-43

[63] Torgerson PR, Abdybekova AM, Minbaeva G, Shapiyeva Z, Thomas LF, Dermauw V, et al. Epidemiology of *Taenia saginata* taeniosis/cysticercosis: A systematic review of the distribution in central and western Asia and the Caucasus. Parasites & Vectors. 2019;**12**(1):175. DOI: 10.1186/s13071-019-3438-3

[64] Lloyd S. Cysticercosis and taeniosis, *Taenia saginata, Taenia solium* and Asian *Taenia*. In: Palmer SRS, LordSimpson DIH, editors. Zoonoses. Oxford, UK: Oxford University Press; 1998. pp. 635-663

[65] Snyder GR, Murrel KD. Bovine cysticercosis. In: Practices in veterinary public health and preventative medicine in U.S.A. Iowa, Ames: Iowa State University Press; 1986;**1**(103):161-170

[66] Wandra T, Sutisna P, Dharmawan NS, Margono SS, Sudewi R, Suroso T, et al. High prevalence of *Taenia saginata* taeniasis and status of *Taenia solium* cysticercosis in Bali, Indonesia, 2002-2004. Transactions of the Royal Society of Tropical Medicine and Hygiene. 2006;**100**(4):346-353. DOI: 10.1016/j.trstmh.2005.06.031

[67] Nakamura Uchiyama F, Hiromatsu K, Ishiwata K, Sakamoto Y, Nawa Y. The current status of parasitic diseases in Japan. Internal Medicine Journal (Tokyo, Japan). 2003;**42**:222-236. DOI: 10.2169/internalmedicine.42.222

[68] Kamiya M, Ooi HK. Current status of foodborne parasitic zoonoses in Japan. The Southeast Asian Journal of Tropical Medicine and Public Health. 1991;**22**:48-53

[69] Bahtia BB. Current status of food-borne parasitic zoonoses in India. The Southeast Asian Journal of Tropical Medicine and Public Health. 1991;**22**:36-41

[70] Edwards SI. Food-borne parasitic zoonoses in the Philippines. The Southeast Asian Journal of Tropical Medicine and Public Health. 1991;**22**:16-22

[71] Ito A et al. Human taeniasis and cysticercosis in Asia. Lancet. 2003;**362**:1918-1920. DOI: 10.1016/S0140-6736(03)14965-3

[72] Parkhouse RME, Harrison LJS. Helminth-cestode: *Taenia saginata* and *Taenia solium*. In: Motarjemi Y, editor. Encyclopedia of Food Safety. Vol. 2. Amsterdam: Academic Press; 2014. pp. 70-77. DOI: 10.1016/B978-0-12-378612-8.00148-7

[73] Ale A, Victor B, Praet N, Gabriël S, Speybroeck N, Dorny P, et al. Epidemiology and genetic diversity of *Taenia asiatica*: a systematic review. Parasites Vectors. 2014;7:45. DOI: 10.1186/1756-3305-7-45

[74] Aung AK, Spelman DW. Taenia solium Taeniasis and Cysticercosis in Southeast Asia. American Journal of Tropical Medicine and Hygiene. 4 May 2016;**94**(5):947-954. DOI: 10.4269/ajtmh.15-0684

[75] Scala A, Varcasia A. Updates on morphobiology, epidemiology and molecular characterization of coenurosis in sheep. Parassitologia. Jun 2006;**48**(1-2):61-63

[76] Varcasia A, Tamponi C, Ahmed F, Cappai MG, Porcu F, Mehmood N, et al. Taenia multiceps coenurosis: A review. Parasit. Vectors. 2022;**15**:1-18. DOI: 10.1186/s13071-022-05210-0

[77] World Health Organization. WHO estimates of the global burden of foodborne diseases: foodborne disease burden epidemiology reference group 2007-2015 (FERG). Geneva: World Health Organization; 2015

[78] García HH, Gonzalez AE, Evans CA, Gilman RH. Cysticercosis Working Group in Peru. Taenia solium cysticercosis. Lancet. 16 Aug 2003;**362**(9383):547-556. DOI: 10.1016/S0140-6736(03)14117-7

[79] Trevisan C, Sotiraki S, Laranjo-González M, et al. Epidemiology of taeniosis/cysticercosis in Europe, a systematic review: Eastern Europe. Parasit. Vectors. 2018;**11**:569. DOI: 10.1186/s13071-018-3153-5

[80] WOAH (World Organisation for Animal Health). Manual of diagnostic tests and vaccines for terrestrial animals. 2022; Part 3, Section 3.4 Bovinae, Chapter 3.4.3 Bovine cysticercosis, Section 3.10 Other diseases, Chapter 3.10.3 Cysticercosis (including infection with *Taenia solium*). Available from: https://www.woah.org/en/what-we-do/standards/codes-and-manuals/terrestrial-manual-online-access/ [Accessed: 2022-12-19]

[81] Directive 2003/99/EC of the European Parliament and of the Council of 17 November 2003 on the monitoring of zoonoses and zoonotic agents, amending Council Decision 90/424/EEC and repealing Council Directive 92/117/EEC, Official Journal of the European Union, L325. 12 Dec 2003. pp. 31-40

[82] EFSA and ECDC (European Food Safety Authority and European Centre for Disease Prevention and Control), 2022. The European Union One Health 2021 Zoonoses Report. EFSA Journal. 2022;**20**(12):7666, 273 pp. DOI: 10.2903/j.efsa.2022.7666

[83] Opinion of the Scientific Panel on Biological Hazards on "Risk assessment of a revised inspection of slaughter animals in areas with low prevalence of Cysticercus". EFSA Journal. 2005;**176**:1-27

[84] Dorny P, Vallée I, Alban L, Boes J, Boireau P, Boué F. et al. Development of harmonised schemes for the monitoring and reporting of Cysticercus in animals and foodstuffs in the European Union. EFSA Suppoting Publication. 2010. DOI: 10.2903/sp.efsa.2010

[85] Dorny P, Brandt J, Geerts S. Chapter 4: Detection and diagnosis. In: Murrell KD, editor. WHO/OIE/FAO guidelines for the surveillance, prevention and control of Taeniosis/Cysticercosis. Paris, France: World Health Organization for Animal Health (OIE); 2005. pp. 45-55

[86] Ostertag R. Handbuch der Fleischbeschau für Tierärzte, Ärzte und Richter. Enke. 1899

[87] Nagel-Alne GE, Murphy E, McCauslin B, Hauge SJ, Schrøder-Petersen DL, Holthe J, et al. Meat safety legislation and its opportunities and hurdles for innovative approaches: A review. Food Control. Nov 2022;**141**:109160. DOI: 10.1016/j.foodcont.2022.109160

[88] Pravilnik o organizaciji službenih kontrola proizvoda životinjskog porijekla namijenjenih ishrani ljudi (in Bosnian language). Official Gazette of Bosnia and Herzegovina, No. 103/2013:66-89

[89] Regulation (EC) No 854/2004 of the European Parliament and of the Council of 29 April 2004 laying down specific rules for the organisation of official controls on products of animal origin intended for human consumption. Official Journal of the European Union, L 30 Apr 2004:206-320

[90] Hill AA, Horigan V, Clarke KA, Dewe TCM, Stärk KDC, O'Brien S, et al. A qualitative risk assessment for visual-only post-mortem meat inspection of cattle, sheep, goats and farmed/wild deer. Food Control. 2014;**38**:96-103. DOI: 10.1016/j.foodcont.2013.10.002

[91] Chalmers RM, Robertson LJ, Dorny P, Jordan S, Kärssin A, Katzer F, et al. Parasite detection in food: Current status and future needs for validation. Trends in Food Science and Technology. 2020;**99**:337-350. DOI: 10.1016/j.tifs.2020.03.011

[92] Jansen F, Dorny P, Berkvens D, Gabriël S. Bovine cysticercosis and taeniosis: The effect of an alternative post-mortem detection method on prevalence and economic impact. Preventive Veterinary Medicine. 1 Dec 2018;**161**:1-8. DOI: 10.1016/j.prevetmed.2018.10.006

[93] Gholami N, Mosayebi M, Dehghan Rahim Abadi P, Rasmi Atigh H, Sedaghat R, Naji Zadeh MH, et al. Bovine cysticercosis in feedlot cattle in central region of Iran. Journal of Parasitic Diseases. Mar 2020;**44**(1):25-30. DOI: 10.1007/s12639-019-01157-9

[94] Kynsgaard NC, Murrell KD. Chapter 5: Prevention of taeniosis and cysticrcosis. In: Murrell KD, editor. WHO/OIE/FAO Guidelines for the Surveillance, Prevention and Control of Taeniosis/Cysticercosis. Paris, France: World Health Organization for Animal Health (OIE); 2005. pp. 57-71

[95] Trevisan C, Mkupasi EM, Ngowi HA, Forkman B, Johansen MV. Severe seizures in pigs naturally infected with *Taenia solium* in Tanzania. Veterinary Parasitology. Apr 2016;**220**:67-71. DOI: 10.1016/j.vetpar.2016.02.025

[96] Prasad KN, Chawla S, Prasad A, Tripathi M, Husain N, Gupta RK. Clinical signs for identification of neurocysticercosis in swine naturally infected with *Taenia solium*. Parasitology International. Jun 2006;**55**(2):151-154. DOI: 10.1016/j.parint.2006.01.002

[97] Mkupasi EM, Ngowi HA, Sikasunge CS, Leifsson PS, Johansen MV. Distribution and histopathological changes induced by cysts of Taenia solium in the brain of pigs from Tanzania. Journal of Helminthology. 6 Jun 2014:1-6. DOI: 10.1017/S0022149X1400042X

[98] Guyatt HL, Fèvre EM. Lingual palpation for porcine cysticercosis: A rapid epidemiological tool for estimating prevalence and community risk in Africa. Tropical Medicine & International Health.

2016;**21**(10):1319-1323. DOI: 10.1111/tmi.12760

[99] Dorny P, Phiri IK, Vercruysse J, Gabriel S, Willingham AL 3rd, Brandt J, et al. A Bayesian approach for estimating values for prevalence and diagnostic test characteristics of porcine cysticercosis. International Journal for Parasitology. Apr 2004;**34**(5):569-576. DOI: 10.1016/j.ijpara.2003.11.014

[100] Sciutto E, Martínez JJ, Villalobos NM, Hernández M, José MV, Beltrán C, et al. Limitations of current diagnostic procedures for the diagnosis of *Taenia solium* cysticercosis in rural pigs. Veterinary Parasitology. Nov 1998;**79**(4):299-313. DOI: 10.1016/s0304-4017(98)00180-0

[101] Kabululu ML, Johansen MV, Mlangwa JED, Mkupasi EM, Braae UC, Trevisan C, et al. Performance of Ag-ELISA in the diagnosis of *Taenia solium* cysticercosis in naturally infected pigs in Tanzania. Parasites & Vectors. 2020;**13**(1):534. DOI: 10.1186/s13071-020-04416-4

[102] Assana E, Kanobana K, Tume CB, Zoli PA, Nguekam, Geerts S, et al. Isolation of a 14 kDa antigen from *Taenia solium* cyst fluid by HPLC and its evaluation in enzyme linked immunosorbent assay for diagnosis of porcine cysticercosis. Research in Veterinary Science. Jun 2007;**82**(3): 370-376. DOI: 10.1016/j.rvsc.2006.09.006

[103] Chembensofu M, Mwape KE, Van Damme I, Hobbs E, Phiri IK, Masuku M, et al. Re-visiting the detection of porcine cysticercosis based on full carcass dissections of naturally *Taenia solium* infected pigs. Parasites & Vectors. 16 Nov 2017;**10**(1):572. DOI: 10.1186/s13071-017-2520-y

[104] Dorny P, Vercammen F, Brandt J, Vansteenkiste W, Berkvens D, Geerts S. Sero-epidemiological study of *Taenia saginata* cysticercosis in Belgian cattle. Veterinary Parasitology. 2000;**88**:43-49. DOI: 10.1016/S0304-4017(99)00196-X

[105] Allepuz A, Gabriël S, Dorny P, Napp S, Jansen F, Vilar MJ, et al. Comparison of bovine cysticercosis prevalence detected by antigen ELISA and visual inspection in the North East of Spain. Research in Veterinary Science. Jun 2012;**92**(3):393-395. DOI: 10.1016/j.rvsc.2011.03.027

[106] Eichenberger RM, Lewis F, Gabriël S, Dorny P, Torgerson PR, Deplazes P. Multi-test analysis and model-based estimation of the prevalence of *Taenia saginata* cysticercus infection in naturally infected dairy cows in the absence of a 'gold standard' reference test. International Journal for Parasitology. Sep 2013;**43**(10):853-859. DOI: 10.1016/j.ijpara.2013.05.011

[107] European Food Safety Authority. Scientific opinion on the public health hazards to be covered by inspection of meat (swine). EFSA Journal. 2011;**9**:2351. DOI: 10.2903/j.efsa.2011.2351

[108] European Food Safety Authority. Scientific opinion on the public health hazards to be covered by inspection of meat from poultry. EFSA Journal. 2012;**10**:2741. DOI: 10.2903/j.efsa.2012.2741

[109] European Food Safety Authority. Scientific Opinion on the public health hazards to be covered by inspection of meat (bovine animals). EFSA Journal. 2013;**11**(6):1e261. DOI: 10.2903/j.efsa.2013.3266

[110] European Food Safety Authority. Technical specifications on harmonised epidemiological indicators for public health hazards to be covered by meat inspection of swine. EFSA Journal.

2011;**9**(10):1-125. DOI: 10.2903/j.efsa.2011.2371

[111] European Food Safety Authority. Technical specifications on harmonised epidemiological indicators for biological hazards to be covered by meat inspection of bovine animals. EFSA Journal. 2013;**11**(6):78. Article ID 3276. DOI: 10.2903/j.efsa.2013.3276

[112] Regulation (EC) No 218/2014 amending annexes to regulation (EC) No 853/2004, (EC), No 854/2004 of the European parliament and of the council and (EC) regulation 2074/2005. OJ L 69. 8 Mar 2014. pp. 95-98

[113] Regulation (EU) 2017/625 of the European Parliament and of the Council of 15 March 2017 on official controls and other official activities performed to ensure the application of food and feed law, rules on animal health and welfare, plant health and plant protection products. OJ L 95. 7 Apr 2017. pp. 1-142

[114] Commission Delegated Regulation (EU) 2019/624 of 8 February 2019 concerning specific rules for the performance of official controls on the production of meat and for production and relaying areas of live bivalve molluscs in accordance with Regulation (EU) 2017/625 of the European Parliament and of the Council. OJ L 131. 17 May 2019. pp. 1-17

[115] Commission Implementing Regulation (EU) 2019/627 laying down uniform practical arrangements for the performance of official controls on products of animal origin intended for human consumption in accordance with Regulation (EU) 2017/625 of the European Parliament and of the Council and amending Commission Regulation (EC) No 2074/2005 as regards official controls. OJ L 131. 17 May 2019. pp. 51-100

[116] Antunović B, Blagojević B, Johler S, Guldimann C, Vieira-Pinto M, Vågsholm I, et al. Challenges and opportunities in the implementation of new meat inspection systems in Europe. Trends Food Science and Technology. 2021;**116**:460-467. DOI: 10.1016/j.tifs.2021.08.002

[117] Blagojevic B, Nesbakken T, Alvseike O, Vågsholm I, Antic D, Johler S, et al. Drivers, opportunities, and challenges of the European risk-based meat safety assurance system. Food Control. 2021;**124**:107870. DOI: 10.1016/j.foodcont.2021.107870

Chapter 3

The Pandemonium of Cysticercosis in Humans

Seljul M.C. Ramyil, Timothy O. Ogundeko, John Bimba, Cornelius S.S. Bello and Amos P. Bassi

Abstract

The pandemonium of cysticercosis in human has pulled the focus of WHO to develop a guideline and promote actions to prevent the causes of epilepsy by taenia worms affecting human health, leading to stigmatization and discrimination and increases public health interventions. In most developing countries such as Sub-Saharan Africa and Asia, cysticercosis mainly affects the health and livelihoods of agrarian farmers, resulting in devastating effects on their health through the ingestion of the parasite's larval cysts in undercooked infected pork or contaminated water. Though, as one of the neglected zoonotic diseases, potentially eradicable yet it is now becoming an emerging disease with approximately 50 million people globally infected.

Keywords: pandemonium, cysticercosis, stigmatization, discrimination, public health interventions, epidemiology

1. Introduction

The World Health Organization foodborne disease burden epidemiology reference group (WHO-FERG) in 2016, estimated and identified the global burden of 31 microorganisms as a leading cause of deaths from foodborne diseases amounting to 2.8 million disability-adjusted life-years (DALY). Because of this, they must be given due consideration as a possible differential diagnosis in areas of high prevalence of cysticercosis, which is termed to be acquired only from the fecal-oral route (ingestion of infected eggs) and ingestion of the cysticerci in undercooked pork that may lead to intestinal taeniasis. The *Taenia solium* tapeworm infections can lead to cysticercosis, which is a disease that can cause seizures, so it is important to seek treatment. In recent times, researchers reported that cysticercosis is prevalent in most West African countries where favorable conditions for parasitic transmission in both humans and pigs occur widely within the region and as such, defecation in the open field, illicit slaughtering of pigs, and unhygienic way of handling meat with unqualified meat inspectors involved in the process [1–3]. The aim of this is to provide updated knowledge as regards cysticercosis diagnostic tools challenges outlined by WHO report in endemic resource-limiting settings and specify needs for adoption to local context considering practical implementation to advance the desire goal for test determinants.

IntechOpen

2. Epidemiology of cysticercosis

The genus Taenia are human parasite consisting of three species (*T. solium*, *T. saginata*, and *T. asiatica*). These parasites live as an adult tapeworms in human intestines causing taeniasis, and the cause leads to cysticercosis in human after ingesting eggs with water, contaminated food, or *via* dirty hands. The World Health Organization (WHO) lists neurocysticercosis as a neglected tropical disease and infection accounted for 50 million people worldwide with 50,000 deaths each year. The clinical manifestations of cysticercosis are highly variable both in kind and in severity with the period of initial infection expressed and the onset of symptoms is generally dependent on the concentration, size, and location of the cysts as well as the host immune response to the parasite's infectivity. However, the preferred locations are the muscles, subcutaneous tissues, central nervous system (CNS), and eyes. Subcutaneous and muscular forms are often asymptomatic. Severe cysticercosis is due to larvae located in human CNS—neurocysticercosis. Most frequently clinical manifestations are seizures, intracranial hypertension, neurological deficits, and sometimes psychiatric manifestations, and over 50% of cases of late-onset epilepsy in developing countries. Usually, cysticercosis is characterized by mild and nonspecific symptoms with abdominal pain, nausea, diarrhea, or constipation may arise when the tapeworms become fully developed in the intestine, approximately 8 weeks after ingestion of meat containing cysticerci. These symptoms may however continue until the tapeworm dies following treatment, otherwise, it may live for several years. In the case of cysticercosis due to *T. solium*, the incubation period prior to the appearance of clinical symptoms is variable, and infected people may remain asymptomatic for many years.

3. The danger of cysticercosis in human

Human cysticercosis can result in devastating effects on human health. The larvae (cysticerci) may develop in the muscles, skin, eyes, and the central nervous system. When cysts develop in the brain, the condition is referred to as neurocysticercosis (NCC). Symptoms include severe headache, blindness, convulsions, and epileptic seizures can be fatal. In developing countries, cysticercosis affects mainly the health and livelihoods of subsistence farmers and reduces the market value of pigs by making the pork unsafe to eat [4, 5].

In developing countries, the endemic human cysticercosis associated with epilepsy is relatively common but rarely reported due to fear of stigmatization. The risk factors for human cysticercosis are closely associated with the characteristics of smallholder or backyard pig farming systems prevalent in this region, which tends to affect poor control and are hampered by infrastructural and financial resources coupled with inadequate information about the eradication and distribution of the disease. The human populations considered to be at the highest risk of infection are those who earn their livelihood wholly or partially through livestock rearing, including pigs, and have limited access to good sanitation [2, 3].

4. Causative agent of cysticercosis in human

The tapeworm Taenia solium invades the human central nervous system and causes neurocysticercosis. The adult tapeworm finds its dwellings in the human small intestine after consumption of varied cysticerci in undercooked pork or contaminated fruits, vegetables, and water, resulting in traceable taeniasis. This zoonotic tapeworm constitutes a serious public health concern as the disease emerged as a continuous problem in most resource-limited settings where pig rearing and pork are served in abundance with little hygienic processes [6]. However, neglected surrounding issues for the presence, magnitude, and parasitic impacts of cysticercosis have led to the disease scarcity of information for the common man [3].

5. Signs and symptoms of cysticercosis in human

Cysticercosis symptoms occurred depending on the site of infection in the human body such that seizures or brain tumor, decreased vision or blindness, abnormal heart rhythms or heart failure and weakness or changes in walking due to damage to the nerves, appearance of lumps under the skin, sometimes vomiting, nausea, headache, dizziness or confusion, and lack of attention resulting in death [7]. Moreso, the antemortem findings present fever in acute stage with muscular stiffness, and the postmortem findings identify cyst in the heart, skeletal muscles, liver, brain, and meninges [8].

6. Complications of cysticercosis in human

The possible complication of cysticercosis may include:

a. Seizures may occur as a result of uncontrolled electrical signals discharged to malfunction the brain cells. This kind of electrical activity overloads the brain functionality causing abnormal sensations and uncontrolled muscle movements [9].

b. Blindness and decreased vision occurred as a result of injuries, inflammation of infections affecting one or two eyes, leading to serious health conditions known as uveitis [9].

7. Diagnostic accuracy of cysticercosis

Diagnostic and management tools for cysticercosis in human resource-limiting settings are challenging in healthcare settings are small, inadequate number of trained personnel, and limited laboratory [10].

It is well documented that the detection of human cysticercosis is key to the management of the disease and identification of proglottids or eggs of *T. solium* have both low sensitivity and specificity, though, a confirmatory of the infection by the adult stage of parasite is made possible macroscopically [11, 12]. However, deoxyribonucleic acid (DNA) based techniques are sensitive and specific [13]. On the other hand, achievable diagnosis of human cysticercosis can be through ELISA, Cysticercus IgG Western Blot Assay, computed tomography (CT) scan, and Magnetic Resonance Imaging (MRI).

8. Sample/specimens appropriate for the diagnosis of cysticercosis

8.1 Noninvasive sampling involving noncritical equipment, materials, and techniques

8.1.1 Fecal specimen

The classic, standard diagnostic tool in most settings is the microscopic examination of stools after concentration with formol-ether aims to demonstrate *Taenia solium* eggs [14]. Moreso, diagnosing taenia tapeworm infection is made by microscopic examination of stool specimen collected on three different days [15].

8.1.2 Urine specimen

Concentration of urine, preparation of *Cysticercus cellulosae* complete homogenate antigen, and hyperimmune cysticercus antiserum were performed by methods described earlier [16, 17].

8.2 Invasive sampling involving critical equipment, materials, and techniques

8.2.1 Cerebrospinal fluid (CSF)

The CSF examination constitutes an important diagnostic and clinical tool in diagnosis of suspected neurocysticercosis [10, 18]. CSF has the advantage of being in more direct contact with the central nervous system (CNS) and its collection requires an aseptic lumber puncture procedure. However, CSF examination may complement serological and biochemical diagnosis. Though, antibody detection by enzyme-linked immunoelectrotransfer blot (EITB) is similarly higher in CSF as compared to other methods [19, 20].

8.2.2 Blood (serum)

Serum samples are preferred for antibody-antigen diagnosis of cysticercosis serologically. Serodiagnostic assay recognized by the World Health Organization and the Pan American Health Organization for cysticercosis and neurocysticercosis outline in Lee et al. [21] in comparison to CSF uses both lentil lectin-purified glycoproteins (LLGP) in an enzyme-linked immunoelectrotransfer blot (EITB) format.

8.2.3 Tissue sampling

Once eggs or proglottids are ingested, oncospheres hatch in the intestine invade the intestinal wall, enter the bloodstream, and migrate to multiple tissues and organs where they mature into cysticerci over several months. Definitive diagnosis consists of the demonstration of the cysticercus in human tissue affected by the larval *Taenia solium* cysts in tissue sections [22].

9. Laboratory diagnosis of human cysticercosis

Diagnosis involves a careful history and physical examination of clinical features, neuroimaging studies [non-computed tomography (CT) scan or Magnetic Resonance

Imaging (MRI)], epidemiological and laboratory-based serological testing in patients strongly suspected of having cysticercosis or neurocysticercosis [22]. In 2015, the WHO report of stakeholder meeting outlined below as diagnostic tools for Taeniasis/Cysticercosis with priorities that this method is time-consuming and requires sophisticated facilities yet in resource-limiting settings, microscopy is necessary at a moment using the formol-ether concentration techniques to demonstrate the visibility of *T. solium* eggs [23].

i. Ag-ELISA, Ab-ELISA, and Corpo-Ag-ELISA: The assay is to perform antigen-antibody glycoprotein embedded enzyme-linked immunosorbent assay (Ag-ELISA) detection in the diagnosis of viable *T. solium* cysticercosis in naturally infected slaughter-age pigs in an endemic area. The Ag-ELISA test characteristics report may indicate that the test is more reliable in ruling out *T. solium* cysticercosis in pigs, than in confirming it [24, 25]. The Ag-ELISA reported a sensitivity range from 86 to 90% and the specificity is estimated at 94–98% the Ab-ELISA reported a specificity of 97.4% and a sensitivity of 96.3% to detect circulating antigens and antibodies in human serum. However, studies indicated that the estimated prevalence rates of human cysticercosis range from 4.6 to 29.7% for Ag-ELISA, and that of Ab-ELISA is reported to be between 1.3 and 51.6% [26] in endemic zones around the world. The estimated prevalence of human cysticercosis antigen around the world is 5.12% and that of the antibodies was estimated to be 15.36%. Nevertheless, these vary from country and region.

ii. LLGP-EITB and EITB: One of the most well-characterized tests for diagnosing neurocysticercosis (NCC) is the enzyme-linked immunoelectrotransfer blot (EITB) assay developed and recommended by CDC uses lentil lectin-bound glycoproteins (LLGP) extracted from *Taenia solium* cysticerci. The test is reliable, but purification process of antigens is difficult to transfer to other laboratories because of expensive nature of the equipment and technical expertise [27]. This has proven to be effective in the detection of neurocysticercosis with 16.7–92.2% prevalence rates with a sensitivity ranging from 97 to 98% and a specificity range from 97 to 100% to detect circulating antibodies to *T. solium* in human serum and considered positive when at least one of the specific glycoproteins from *T. solium* metacestodes is recognized by the serum [28].

iii. Copro-PCR (Multiplex, Nested, and RT-PCR): Multiplex, Nested, and Real-Time PCR assay is developed to target *Tso31* gene for specific diagnosis of cysticercosis due to *T. solium*. The estimated sensitivity of this test was reported to be 82.7% with a specificity of 99% for real-time polymerase chain reaction assay (copro-PCR) 99% (95% CI: [98.2–99.6]) for copro-PCR [29]. These methods are more sensitive than microscopy but cross-react with *T. saginata*. However, the differentiation of *T. solium* and *T. saginata* is based on the morphological characteristics of the scolex or gravid proglottids [30].

iv. Microscopy: Human intestinal infectivity with adult *T. solium* worms can be diagnosed by microscopic examination of stool samples and identification of ova or proglottids are present in ≤50% of stool samples from patients with cysticercosis, which has very low sensitivity and specificity [31].

10. Prevention, control, and treatment of cysticercosis

10.1 Mass treatment

Mass treatment of human decreases logistic costs and increases feasibility with high-advantage interventions around the geohelminths regions requiring less field visits and concern raised about environmental contamination [14].

10.2 Community health education

Health education of the target population most captured educational design of control/elimination programs to increase sustainability. Individuals without knowledge of infected meat have a higher risk of getting taeniasis by mis-ingestion and may subsequently get cysticercosis [32]. Community education in combination with a multipronged approach consisting of vaccination of pigs is necessary.

10.3 Targeted treatment of infected persons

Targeted treatment is effective to decrease the source of infection, finding infected individuals with informed intervention choice of treatment and drug optimization.

10.4 Meat radiation and freezing

The use of gamma-radiation and meat freezing for more than 1–3 days as proposed by Verster et al. [33] and Sotelo et al. [34] killed cysts before pork consumption and minimized the use of expensive and sophisticated equipment discussed in Gilman et al. [14].

10.5 Personal hygiene

Personal hygiene and sanitary health measures are critical to avoid human feco-oral contamination where indiscriminate defecations are identified as a risk factor for cysticercosis. Individuals with such poor defecating habits generally have poor hygienic behaviors and thereby increase the high risk of cysticercosis. Regular handwashing with soap and running tap water, proper washing of fruits, vegetables before eating, and washing of cutleries/utensils reduces the risk of infectivity [3, 10, 32, 35] (**Table 1**).

10.6 Treatment

Cysticercosis if treated include immediate measures to prevent morbidity and mortality, and following surgical to control seizures, corticosteroids to control inflammation, and anthelminthic medications to kill cysts as outlined below:

i. Corticosteroids (Prednisolone, Dexamethasone) are disintegrated tables used to treat and reduce inflammatory bowel disease conditions and adrenal gland disorders.

ii. Antiepileptic/Anticonvulsant medications (Phenytoin, carbamazepine) to reduce and prevent the risk of seizures.

iii. Antiparasitic medications (Albendazole, Praziquantel) are often used to kill cyst infections.

iv. Surgery to removal of cysts or to put in a tube to redirect the fluids in the brain induced by the presence of cysticerci.

Globally, studies for circulating human cysticercosis antigen were 5.52% in positive cases and 14.20% for antibodies. Although, the incessant use of pig feces

Country or region	Assay	Percentage (%)	Reference
Latin America	Ag-ELISA	0.94–9.12	Coral-Almeida et al. [26]
	Ab-ELISA or EITB	1.82–31.22	Bruno et al. [36]
Asia	Ag-ELISA	15.7–41.8	Ar Kar et al. [37]
	Ab-ELISA	4.0–26.7	Coral-Almeida et al. [26]
	EITB	46.7–66.7	Bizhani et al. [38]
Africa	Ag-ELISA	0.7–21.63	Gulelat et al. [39]
	Ab-ELISA	1.3–45.3	Coral-Almeida et al. [26]
	EITB	6.9–16.7	Shonyela et al. [29]
	CT Scan	23.2–54.6	Praet et al. [40]
	Copro-PCR (or Copro-ELISA)	5.2–14.8	Praet et al. [40]
West Africa	Ag-ELISA	4.6–11.9	Shonyela et al. [29], Weka et al. [41]
	Ab-ELISA or EITB	24.7–51.6	Edia-Asuke et al. [42]
Nigeria	Ab-ELISA or EITB	9.6–14.3	Weka et al. [41]

Table 1.
The global estimated prevalence rates of human cysticercosis.

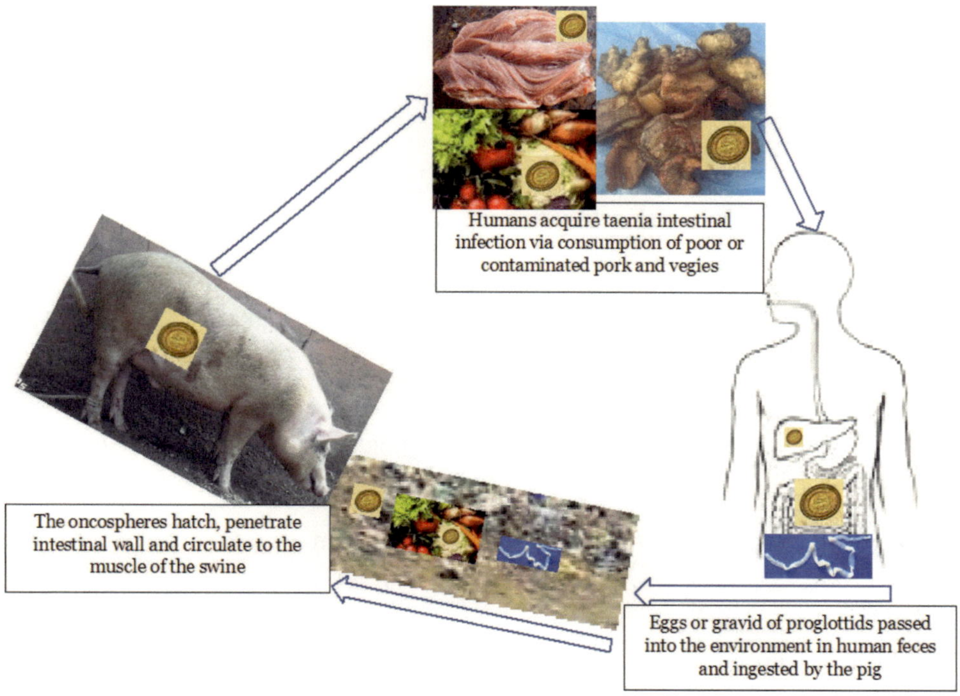

Figure 1.
Life cycle of Taenia solium (human cysticercosis).

as fertilizer has become imperative to farmers and poses the risk of cysticerci food contamination, thereby supporting encystment. However, heavy infectivity calls for the carcass's complete condemnation despite the provision for freezing treatment, though pending approval in light or moderate infestation (**Figure 1**).

11. Conclusion

Despite WHO having focused on developing a policy and promoting measures to avoid the cause of seizures by Taenia/Cysticercosis impacting human health, leading to stigmatization and increasing public initiatives because of the challenges of human cysticercosis. The increasing risk of human cysticercosis in developing countries is reported to be significantly associated with the consumption of the parasites' cysts in raw, infected pork, or contaminated food and water. Understanding the epidemiology of human cysticercosis will help to expose critical information about the transmission of the disease, thereby intensifying efforts for effective low assessable control and prevention measures.

Declaration of interest

We declared that there is no conflict of interest whatsoever that could affect this work, leading to bias but recognized the materials used in this article are well cited and referenced appropriately.

Author details

Seljul M.C. Ramyil*, Timothy O. Ogundeko, John Bimba, Cornelius S.S. Bello and Amos P. Bassi
College of Medicine and Allied Health Sciences, Bingham University Jos Campus, Nigeria

*Address all correspondence to: crownramyil@yahoo.com

IntechOpen

© 2023 The Author(s). Licensee IntechOpen. This chapter is distributed under the terms of the Creative Commons Attribution License (http://creativecommons.org/licenses/by/3.0), which permits unrestricted use, distribution, and reproduction in any medium, provided the original work is properly cited.

References

[1] Weka RP, Kamani J, Cogan T, Eisler M, Morgan ER. Overview of Taenia solium cysticercosis in West Africa. Acta Tropica. 2019;**190**:329-338. DOI: 10.1016/j.actatropica.2018.12.012. Available from: https://www.sciencedirect.com/science/article/pii/S0001706X18310660

[2] Carabin H et al. Prevalence of and factors associated with human cysticercosis in 60 villages in three Provinces of Burkina Faso. PLoS Neglected Tropical Diseases. 2015;**9**(11):e0004248. DOI: 10.1371/journal.pntd.0004248

[3] WHO (2016). Taenia Solium Taeniasis/Cysticercosis Diagnostic Tools: Report of a Stakeholder Meeting, Geneva. WHO/HTM/NTD/NZD/2016.4; 2015. p. 16

[4] Proaño-Narvaez JV, Meza-Lucas A, Mata-Ruiz O, García-Jerónimo RC, Correa D. Laboratory diagnosis of human neurocysticercosis: Double-blind comparison of enzyme-linked immunosorbent assay and electroimmunotransfer blot assay. Journal of Clinical Microbiology. 2002;**40**(6):2115-2118. DOI: 10.1128/JCM.40.6.2115-2118.2002

[5] WHO. 2022 Taenia Solium-use of Existing Diagnostic Tools in Public Health Programmes: Report of Virtual Meeting of Experts. Geneva: WHO. Licence: CC BY-NC_SA 3.0IGO; 2022

[6] Johansen MV et al. Are we ready for Taenia solium cysticercosis elimination in sub-Saharan Africa? Parasitology. 2017;**144**(1):59-64. DOI: 10.1017/S0031182016000500

[7] CDC. Following the diagnostic development pathway to better health. World Neglected Tropical Diseases. 2023:2023. Available from: www.cdc.gov/parasites.CS329448-BA

[8] Jackson GJ. USA in Manual on Meat Inspection for Developing Countries, Chapter 4 Specific Diseases of Pigs. Washington D.C.: Division of Microbiology, US FDA. Available from: https://www.fao.org/3/t0756e/T0756E05.htm

[9] Cleveland clinic.org. Cysticercosis: Overview, Symptoms and Treatment. 2022. 23534-cysticercosis

[10] Butala C, Brook TM, Majekodunmi AO, Welburn SC. Neurocysticercosis: Current perspective on diagnosis and management. Frontiers in Veterinary Science. 2021;**8**:615703. DOI: 10.3389/Fvets.2021.615703

[11] Nkwengulila G. A review of human cysticercosis and diagnostic challenges in endemic resource poor countries. Advances in Infectious Diseases. 2014;**4**:207-213. DOI: 10.4236/aid.2014.44029

[12] Rodriguez S, Wilkins P, Dorny P. Immunological and molecular diagnosis of cysticercosis. Global Health Pathway. 2012;**106**:286-298

[13] Gonza'leza LM, Monteroa E, Puenteb S, Lo'pez-Velezc R, Herna'ndezd M, Sciuttod S, et al. PCR tools for the differential diagnosis of *Taenia saginata* and *Taenia solium* taeniasis/cysticercosis from different geographical locations. Diagnostic Microbiology and Infectious Disease. 2002;**42**(2002):243-249. Available from: http://www.elsevier.com/locate/diagmicrobio

[14] Gilman RH, Gonzalez AE, Llanos-Zavalaga F, Tsang VC, Garcia HH,

Cysticercosis Working Group in Peru. Prevention and control of *Taenia solium* taeniasis/cysticercosis in Peru. Pathogens and Global Health. 2012;**106**(5):312-318. DOI: 10.1179/2047773212Y.0000000045

[15] Marie C, William A, Petri Jr. *Taenia solium* (Pork Tapeworm) Infection and Cysticercosis University of Virginia School of Medicine Last review/revision Dec 2021 Modified Sep 2022. Rahway, NJ, USA: Merck & Co, Inc.; 2022. (known as MSD outside the US and Canada). Available from: https://www.msdmanuals.com/professional/infectious-diseases/cestodes-tapeworms/taenia-solium-pork-tapeworm-infection-and-cysticercosis

[16] Biswas R, Parija SC. Latex agglutination test for the detection of cysticercus antigen in the urine for the diagnosis of neurocysticercosis. Tropical Parasitology. 2013;**3**(2):168-169. DOI: 10.4103/2229-5070.122152

[17] Parija M, Biswas R, Harish BN, Parija SC. Detection of specific cysticercus antigen in the urine for diagnosis of neurocysticercosis. Acta Tropica. 2004;**92**:253-260

[18] Bazan R, Odashima NS, Luvizutto GJ, Filho PTH, Zanini MA, Takayanagui OM. Analysis of cerebrospinal fluid in racemose form of neurocysticercosis. Arquivos de Neuro-Psiquiatria. 2015;**73**(10):852-855. DOI: 10.1590/0004-282X20150120 doi:10.1590/0004-282X20150120

[19] Bueno EC, Jose' Vaz A, LDR M, Livramento JA, Mielle SR. Specific taenia crassiceps and taenia solium antigenic peptides for neurocysticercosis immunodiagnosis using serum samples. Journal of Clinical Microbiology. 2000;**38**(1):146-151. Available from: https://journals.asm.org/journal/jcm

[20] Garcia HH, O'Neal SE, Noh J, Handali S, Cysticercosis Working Group in Peru. Laboratory diagnosis of neurocysticercosis (*Taenia solium*). Journal of Clinical Microbiology. 2018;**56**(9):e00424-e00418. DOI: 10.1128/JCM.00424-18

[21] Lee Y-M, Sukwan H, Kathy H, Sowmya P, Victor KA, Andrew L, et al. Serologic diagnosis of human *Taenia solium* cysticercosis by using recombinant and synthetic antigens in QuickELISA™. American Journal of Tropical Medicine and Hygiene. 2011;**84**(4):587-593. DOI: 10.4269/ajtmh.2011.10-0079

[22] CDC, Parasite_Cysticercosis _Biology 2021. Available from: https://www.cdc.gov/parasites/cysticercosis/biology

[23] WHO. Estimates of the Global Burden of Foodnorne Diseases. Foodborne Disease Burden Epidemiology Reference Group 2007 – 2015. Geneva: WHO; 2015. p. 2015. Available from: http://www.who.int/foodssafety/publications/food-borne.disease/fergreport/en/

[24] Kabululu ML, Johansen MV, Mlangwa JED, et al. Performance of Ag-ELISA in the diagnosis of *Taenia solium* cysticercosis in naturally infected pigs in Tanzania. Parasites Vectors. 2020;**13**:534. DOI: 10.1186/s13071-020-04416-4

[25] Arroyo G, Rodriguez S, Ag L, Alroy KA, Bustes JA, Santivanez S. Antibody banding patterns of the enzyme-linked immunoelectransfer blot and brain imaging finding in patients with neurocysticercosis. Clinical Infectious Diseases. 2018;**2018**(66):282-288. DOI: 101093/cid774

[26] Coral-Almeida M, Gabriël S, Abatih EN, Praet N, Benitez W, Dorny P. *Taenia solium* human

cysticercosis: A systematic review of sero-epidemiological data from endemic zones around the world. PLoS Neglected Tropical Diseases. 2015;**9**:e0003919. DOI: 10.1371/journal.pntd.0003919

[27] Noh J, Rodriguez S, Lee YM, Handali S, Gonzalez AE, Gilman RH, et al. Recombinant protein- and synthetic peptide-based immunoblot test for diagnosis of neurocysticercosis. Journal of Clinical Microbiology. 2014;**52**(5):1429-1434. DOI: 10.1128/JCM.03260-13

[28] Rahantamalala A, Rakotoarison RL, Rakotomalala E, Rakotondrazaka M, Kiernan J, Castle PM, et al. Prevalence and factors associated with human *Taenia solium* taeniosis and cysticercosis in twelve remote villages of Ranomafana rainforest, Madagascar. PLOS Neglected Tropical Diseases. 2022;**16**(4):e0010265. DOI: 10.1371/journal.pntd.0010265

[29] Shonyela SM, Yang GL, Wang CF. Current status of prevalence, possible control and risk factors associated with porcine cysticercosis from endemic countries in Africa. World Journal of Vaccines. 2018;**8**:53-80. DOI: 10.4236/wjv.2018.83006

[30] Mayta H, Gilman RH, Prendergast E, Castillo JP, Tinoco YO, Garcia HH, et al. Nested PCR for specific diagnosis of *Taenia solium* taeniasis. Journal of Clinical Microbiology. 2008;**46**(1):286-289. DOI: 10.1128/JCM.01172-07

[31] Al-Awadhi M, Iqbal J, Ahmad S. Cysticercosis, a potential public health concern in kuwait: A new diagnostic method to screen taenia solium taeniasis carriers in the expatriate population. Medical Principles and Practice: International Journal of the Kuwait University, Health Science Centre. 2020;**29**(4):347-353. DOI: 10.1159/000504625

[32] Cao W, Der V, PLoeg CPB, Xu J, Gao C, Ge L, et al. Risk factors for human cysticercosis morbidity: A populationbased case-control study. Epidemiology and Infection. 1997;**119**:231-235

[33] Verster A, Du Plessis TA, van Den Heever LW. The effect of gamma radiation on the cysticerci of *Taenia solium*. The Onderstepoort Journal of Veterinary Research. 1976;**43**(1):23-26

[34] Sotelo J, Rosas N, Palencia G. Freezing of infested pork muscle kills cysticerci. Journal of the American Medical Association. 1986;**256**(7):893-894

[35] Srikanth S, Anandam G. Cysticercosis: The day to day public health problem and the various sites affected by it—A one year study. Tropical Parasitology. 2013;**3**(2):132-134. DOI: 10.4103/2229-5070.122133

[36] Bruno E, Bartoloni A, Zammarchi L, Strohmeyer M, Bartalesi F, Bustos JA, et al. Epilepsy and neurocysticercosis in Latin America: A systematic review and meta-analysis. PLoS Neglected Tropical Diseases. 2013;**7**(10):e2480. DOI: 10.1371/journal.pntd.0002480

[37] Aung AK, Spelman DW. *Taenia solium* taeniasis and cysticercosis in southeast Asia: A review. American Journal of Tropical Medicine and Hygiene. 2016;**94**(5):947-954. DOI: 10.4269/ajtmh.15-0684

[38] Bizhani N, Hashemi Hafshejani S, Mohammadi N, Rezaei M, Rokni MB. Human cysticercosis in Asia: A systematic review and meta-analysis. Iranian Journal of Public Health. 2020;**49**(10):1839-1847. DOI: 10.18502/ijph.v49i10.4683

[39] Gulelat Y, Eguale T, Kebede N, Aleme H, Fèvre EM, Cook EAJ.

Epidemiology of porcine cysticercosis in eastern and southern Africa: Systematic review and meta-analysis. Frontiers in Public Health. 2022;**10**:836177. DOI: 10.3389/fpubh.2022.836177

[40] Praet N, Verweij JJ, Mwape KE, Phiri IK, Muma JB, Zulu G, et al. Bayesian modelling to estimate the test characteristics of coprology, coproantigen ELISA and a novel real-time PCR for the diagnosis of taeniasis. Tropical Medicine & International Health. 2013;**18**(5):608-614

[41] Weka R, Luka P, Ogo N, Weka P. Taenia solium cysticercosis in pigs and human: A review of epidemiological data in West Africa (1990-2019). IntechOpen. 2020. DOI: 10.5772/intechopen.89559

[42] Edia-Asuke AU, Inabo HI, Mukaratirwa S, Umoh VJ, Whong CM, Asuke S, et al. Seroprevalence of human cysticercosis and its associated risk factors among humans in areas of Kaduna metropolis, Nigeria. Journal of Infection in Developing Countries. 2015;**9**:799-805

Chapter 4

Taenia solium Taeniasis and Cysticercosis Prevalence and Control Practice in China

Junqiang Li and Longxian Zhang

Abstract

Taenia solium taeniasis/cysticercosis is an important global food-borne zoonosis transmitted between humans and pigs. In China, the prevalence of *Theridion solium* taeniasis/cysticercosis has been marked decline in recent decades based on the data revealed by both national surveys and field prevalence investigations. Health education and promotion, meat inspection, and chemotherapy are unquestionably the main control measures for diseases. It is worth noting that a variety of socio-ecological variables have been identified in the process of controlling *T. solium* taeniasis/cysticercosis. It has become difficult for pigs to come into direct or indirect contact with or consume human excreta as pig farming practices have been shifted from traditional backyard farms to large-scale commercial pig raising systems that are still in progress. The human toilet revolution in rural areas of China has ensured hygienic separation of human excreta from contact, and thereby preventing human excreta from polluting the soil, feeds, and water. These two important fundamental preventive measures are crucial to establishing an environmental restriction between humans and pigs cannot be overlooked for interrupting or limiting *T. solium* transmission. In this chapter, we reviewed the epidemiology, traditional measures, and ecological determinants that significantly contributed to the dramatic decline of taeniasis/cysticercosis in China.

Keywords: *Taenia solium*, epidemiology, control, ecological determinants, China

1. Introduction

Taenia solium taeniasis/cysticercosis is an important food-borne zoonosis which is transmitted between humans and pigs all over the world [1, 2]. Taeniasis typically causes several digestive problems in humans, whereas cysticercosis is a very serious disease in both humans and pigs [3]. Porcine cysticercosis primarily parasitizes muscle tissues and visceral organs throughout the body of pig resulting in poor quality of pork. However, human cysticercosis may take several pathological forms such as neurocysticercosis (NCC), ocular cysticercosis (OCC), subcutaneous muscle cysticercosis, oral cavity cysticercosis, visceral cysticercosis, and others [3–5]. Human NCC is mainly responsible for seizures, high intracranial pressure, and psychiatric disorders, and it is considered to be one of the major disease burdens in people in many parts of the world [6].

IntechOpen

Theridion solium taeniasis/cysticercosis is a severe helminth infection common in humans and domestic pigs raised in close proximity to human settlements, particularly those in warm and mild climates in Latin America, Sub-Saharan Africa, Southeast Asia, the Indian subcontinent, and China [7–9]. In some endemic areas of *T. solium*, cysticercosis is a leading cause of epileptic seizures in humans [10, 11], while NCC has been noticed as a health burden even in non-endemic regions such as America and Europe owing to frequent traveling and immigration [2, 12]. Approximately 50 million people worldwide suffer from NCC caused by *T. solium* with more than 50,000 deaths per year [13], and studies have indicated a higher prevalence of cysticercosis and its burden than has been recognized by the public health service systems [14, 15].

As the life cycle of *T. solium* involves humans and pigs (**Figure 1**), humans acquire tapeworm infection by consuming raw or under-cooked pork containing cysticerci [16]. Following ingestion, the larval tapeworm grows into an adult worm within approximately 2 months in the human small intestine [16]. Humans are the only natural definitive hosts who harbor the adult form of *T. solium* in their small intestines [8]. Eggs or the most distal worm segments (proglottids) containing mature eggs are released as they frequently detach from the worm and then are passed out into the environment with human feces [8, 17]. These eggs can infect the same (auto-infection) or other humans through fecal-oral transmission from direct contact with tapeworm carriers or consumption of water or food contaminated with human feces [6, 16, 18]. Pigs acquire infection through consumption of human feces containing infectious eggs (gravid proglottids) as well as contaminated food, water, and soil [8]. Humans and pigs could both serve as intermediate hosts, and the embryo (oncosphere) is released after ingestion and migrates through the intestinal mucosa. Later, the larval stages (cysticerci) lead to systemic infection in brain, eyes, subcutaneous tissues, and viscera of the host *via* blood circulatory system [8].

Domestication of wild boars (*Sus scrofa*) began 9000 years ago, and pig rearing has been a common practice in Asian countries for more than 2500 years [19]. Cysticercosis has long been a worldwide zoonosis transmitted between pigs and humans [3]. In China, the prevalence of *T. solium* taeniasis/cysticercosis has been significantly reduced in the recent decades as a result of ongoing health education and promotion as well as sanitary improvements [3, 20, 21]. There have been noticeably dramatic changes in pig-rearing methods and socio-ecological factors as well in China [22, 23]. In this chapter, we reviewed the epidemiology, traditional measures, and ecological determinants that outstandingly contributed to the decline of *T. solium* taeniasis/cysticercosis in China.

2. Epidemiological records

2.1 National surveys on human taeniasis/cysticercosis

Three national surveys on parasitic diseases in humans have been conducted in China until now (**Table 1**). In the first national survey (1988–1992), a total of 1,477,742 individuals from 30 out of 34 provinces in China were investigated, and 2449 individuals from 28 provinces were found to have *Taenia* spp. infections [24]. These data led to an estimation of about 1.3 million cases of *Taenia* spp. infection in the country [25]. The second nationwide survey (2001–2004) conducted in 31 provinces (out of 34 provinces in China) with a total sample size of 356,629 people revealed that 983 people from 12 provinces (38.7%, 12/31) were diagnosed to have *Taenia* spp. infestation [26]. According to these findings, 0.55 million people were infected in total estimation [26].

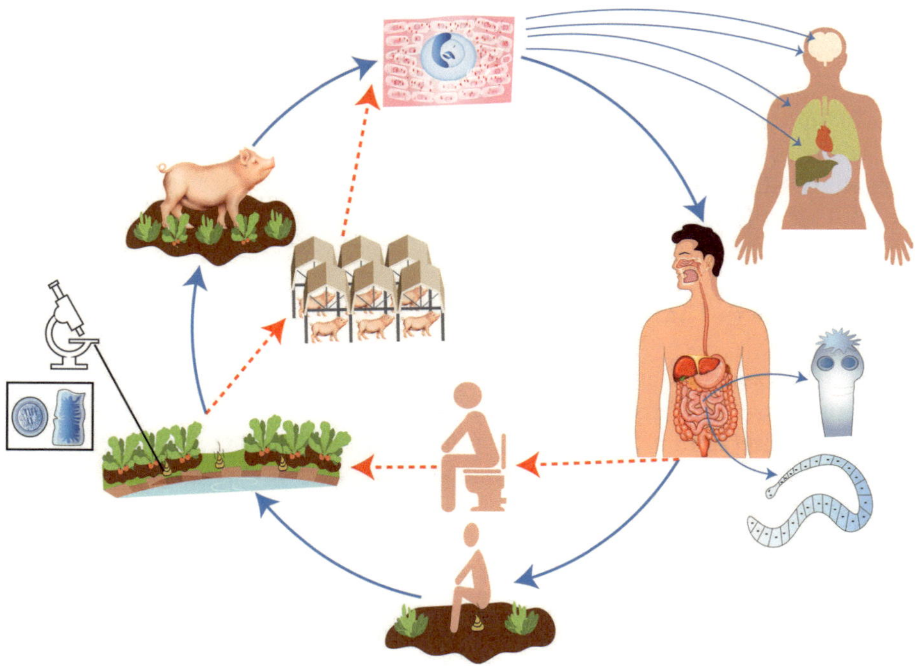

Figure 1.
The life cycle and mode of transmission of Taenia solium in humans and pigs. The blue cycle indicates the traditional life cycle of Taenia solium. Humans become infected and the tapeworms colonize in the gut after consuming raw or undercooked pork containing larval tapeworm, the cysticerci that matures into an adult worm in the human small intestine in about 2 months. The worm's eggs or the most distal segments (proglottids) carrying mature eggs are periodically released/detached and subsequently discharged into the environment with human stool. Pigs get infected when they consume infectious eggs (gravid proglottids) in human excrement, food, water, and soil. Both humans and pigs could serve as intermediate hosts, and the embryo (oncosphere) is released after ingestion and migrates through the intestinal mucosa. Later, the larval stages (cysticercus) commonly infest host body organs such as the brain, eyes, subcutaneous tissues, and viscera via the blood circulatory system. Similarly, humans become infected by consuming raw or undercooked pork containing cysticerci that mature into an adult worm in the small intestine in about 2 months. The red dashed cycle represents the rebuilding Theridion solium life cycle. As a result of a structural shift in pig farming from backyard to large-scale intensive pig farming, as well as a toilet revolution aimed at improving sanitary conditions, the transmission of T. solium between humans and pigs has been significantly interrupted, and spread of the disease is being gradually lessened.

Surveys	Sampling periods	Number of provinces surveyed/ total number of participants	Positive provinces/ participants	Estimated prevalence in whole nation	Estimated infection cases in whole nation
First	1988–1992	30/1,477,742	28/2449	0.17%	1.3 million
Second	2001–2004	31/356,629	12/983	0.28%	0.55 million
Third	2014–2015	31/617,441	12/1752	0.06%[a]	0.37 million

[a]*It was a weighted prevalence, and it was estimated after adjustment by the population structure in total population.*

Table 1.
National surveys on human taeniasis/cysticercosis in China.

Likewise, in the third nationwide survey (2014–2015), *Taenia* spp. was found in 1752 people from 12 provinces (38.7%, 12/31) out of 617,441 people under investigation from 31 provinces (out of 34 provinces in China) [27]. Considering the demographic structure in the whole population, a weighted prevalence of 0.06 percent was calculated, implying that 0.37 million people were infected [27].

Three national surveys on human parasitic disease in China revealed a significant decline in human *T. solium* taeniasis/cysticercosis, while recorded cases indicated that *T. solium* cysticercosis was traditionally endemic in northeastern, central, and southwestern China (**Figure 2**). However, infection rates have been high in areas in the southwest of China with poor socioeconomic conditions, particularly in Tibet, Sichuan, and Yunnan [3, 28–30].

2.2 Case summary of human taeniasis/cysticercosis

There are a variety of human taeniasis/cysticercosis case reports in China. Among them, brain neurocysticercosis (NCC) was the most prevalent (75.87%), followed by subcutaneous infections (11.17%). Several reports have documented mixed infections related to multiple organs, with the brain and subcutaneous cysticercosis being the most common (4.74%) (**Figure 3**).

2.3 Prevalence of human taeniasis/cysticercosis

The epidemiology of human taeniasis/cysticercosis has been well documented and recorded in the same area for many years (**Figure 4A**). It is observed that the prevalence rates have generally been declining when the prevalence rates for various years in the same location are compared [3, 28, 29]. Analysis of risk factors revealed that the prevalence of human cysticercosis is the highest in areas where sanitation is poor, toilets are lacking, and people traditionally consume raw or under-cooked pork (or viscera) and/or where pig husbandry is substandard [3, 28, 29, 31–33].

2.4 Field prevalence of porcine cysticercosis

As with human cysticercosis, there were numerous studies on the epidemiology of porcine cysticercosis, which were mostly carried out during the slaughter quarantine. For a comparative analysis of the prevalence rates of the human cysticercosis for different years in the same area, it is found that the prevalence has been significantly declining (**Figure 4B**). Humans are the only natural definitive host for cysticercosis [8], and pigs become infected through consumption of human feces in areas where open human defecation is common, and also through contaminated food, water, and soil [8].

3. Traditional control measures

3.1 Health education and promotion

As with other infectious diseases, the transmission of *T. solium* taeniasis/cysticercosis requires three key links, such as infectious source, route of transmission, and susceptible population which are correlated [21]. Health education and promotion primarily target the susceptible population and infected individuals (**Table 2**). In view of the serious harm to human health and animal husbandry for taeniasis and cysticercosis of swine, the "Qu Tao Mie Nang" movement had been extensively carried out in the endemic areas from 1970s to 1990s in Chinese mainland.

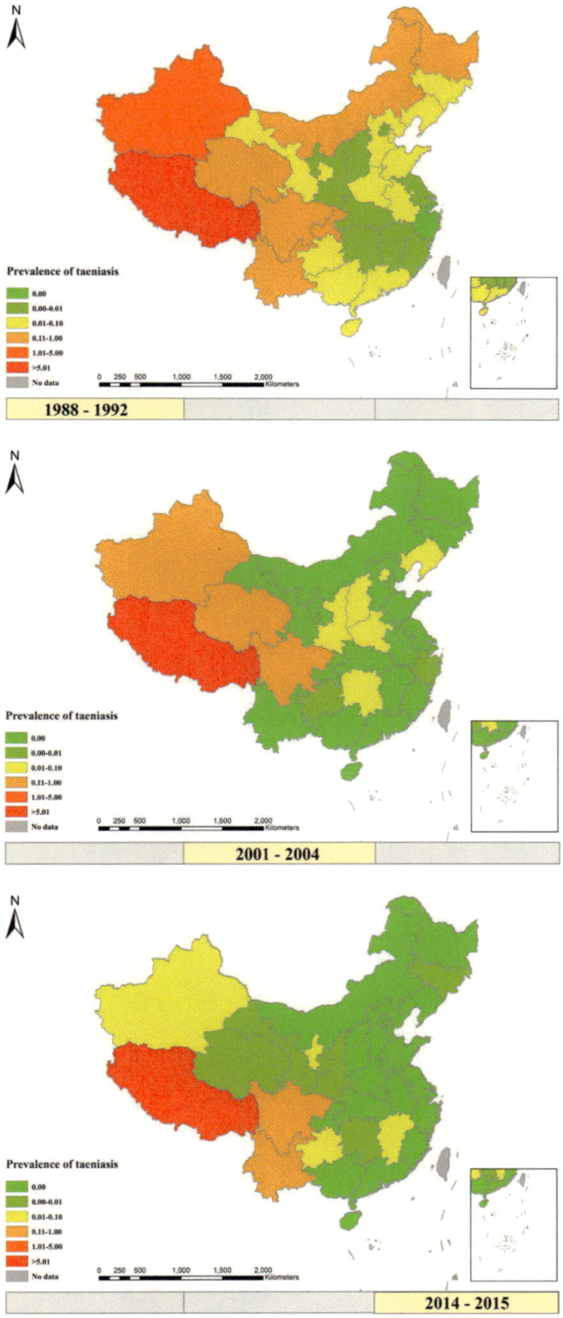

Figure 2.
Three national surveys on human taeniasis/cysticercosis in China (adapted from [3]). Different colors represent different prevalence of taeniasis during three national surveys. The darker color (red) indicates the higher prevalence rate, and the lighter color (green) indicates the lower prevalence rate. Theridion solium cysticercosis was historically prevalent in northeastern, southwestern, and central China, and three national surveys claimed that the frequency of taeniasis has decreased considerably in most areas of China. However, infections have been high in areas of Southwest China with poor socioeconomic conditions, particularly in Chinese Tibet, Sichuan, and Yunnan.

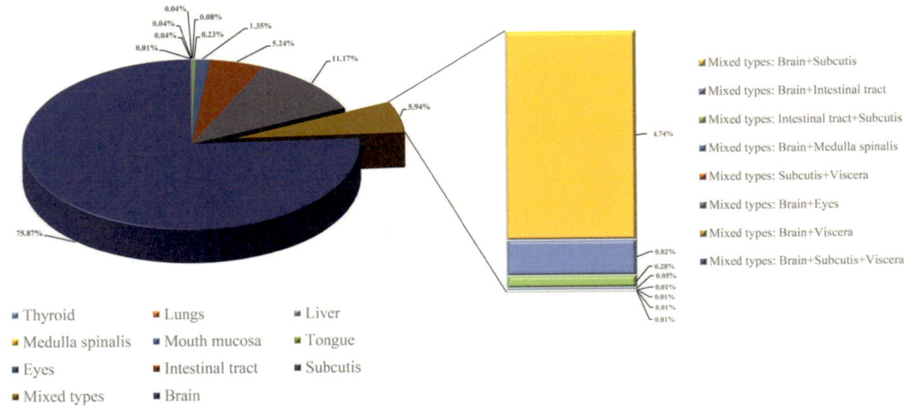

Figure 3.
Case records from hospitalized patients with taeniasis/cysticercosis in China.

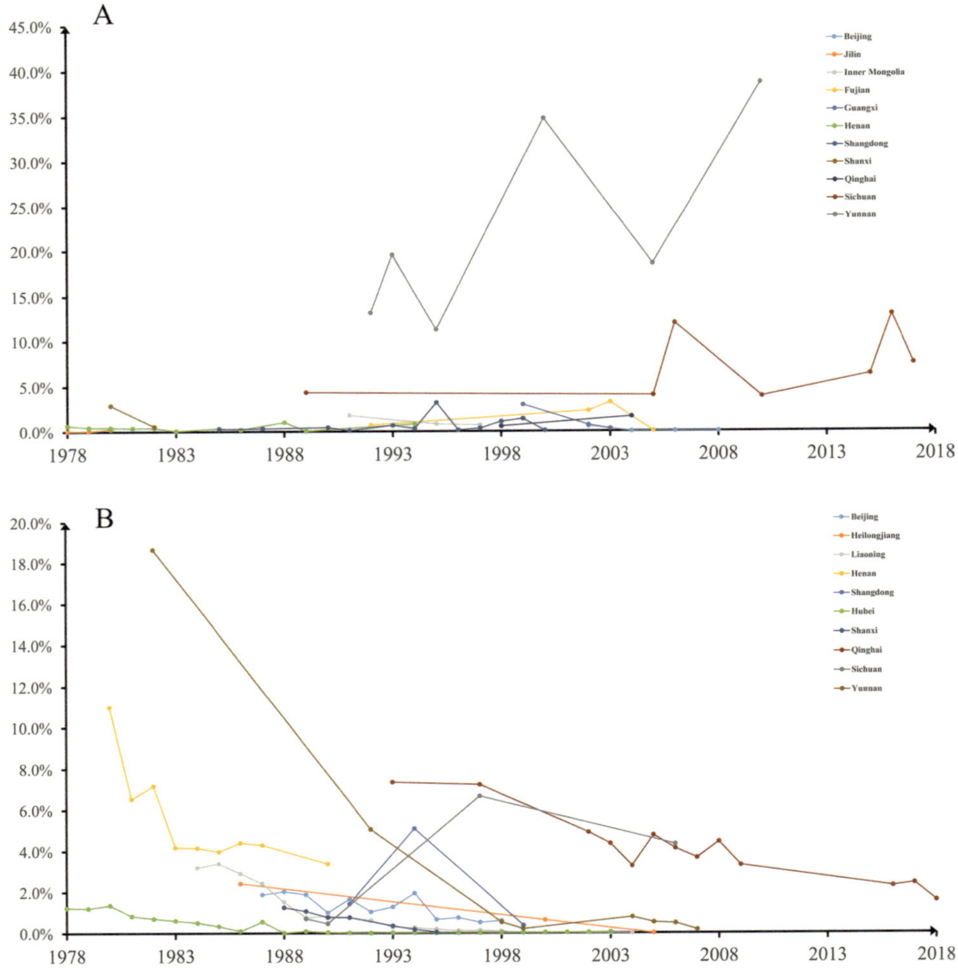

Figure 4.
Field prevalence investigations of human taeniasis/cysticercosis (a) and porcine cysticercosis (b) in the past decades by regional distributions. The prevalence of porcine cysticercosis has been noticeably declining, according to a comparison of the documented cases during the slaughter quarantine for various years in the same region.

Serial number	Main content
1st	Keep the human toilet and pigsty separate, and keep the pigpen clean
2nd	Avoid pigs eating human stool or contaminated feeds and water
3rd	Strengthen slaughter quarantine of pigs, prohibit the sale of pork with cysticercosis, and use harmless treatment
4th	Do not eat raw pork or pig skins
5th	Treatment in time if got sick

Table 2.
Health education and promotion for Theridion solium taeniasis/cysticercosis in China (adapted from [34]).

The main objective of the movement was the treatment of the human taeniasis and elimination of pig cysticercosis. The strategy of the same movement was the early treatment of taeniasis in patients once diagnosed, carry out extensive pork quarantine in urban and rural areas to ensure the quality of meat products, speed up the transformation of rural toilets, and improve the environmental sanitation to obstacle the disease transmission routes, and treatment of human patients and pigs with cysticercosis with the application of effective drugs. It refers to a comprehensive social and political process that includes not only improving individual knowledge, lifestyle, and life skills, but also changing societal, environmental, and economic conditions to reduce the negative effects of parasitism on individuals and communities [20, 21].

3.2 Meat inspection

Pork contaminated with cysticercus is a major source of human *T. solium* taeniasis and cysticercosis transmission. Inspection of pork at slaughter is an important public health measure to prevent the transmission of *T. solium* to humans [16]. However, meat inspection is usually only effective in detecting heavily infected carcasses and is not much reliable in detecting lightly infected carcasses because it depends on the expertise of the meat inspector [35]. Cysticerci can be confused with sarcocystis, milk spots, hydatid cysts, and even unstructured fat and muscle fasciae [35, 36].

Unfortunately, in some parts of China, national pork inspection guidelines are insufficient for detecting cysticercosis. In particular, illegal slaughters occur frequently when pigs are suspected of having cysticercosis in order to avoid economic loss due to the fear of infected pigs likely to be confiscated [16]. Another example is the consumption of raw or under-cooked pork as a traditional way of life in some areas, particularly in/from Sichuan, Yunnan, and Guangxi, China, where pigs are raised in substandard conditions [28, 30, 31, 33, 37, 38]. These days, great strides have been made in health education and promotion.

3.3 Chemotherapy

For the current chemotherapy, it is now possible to actively identify and treat parasite-infected patients, and even to perform mass chemotherapy due to the availability of effective anthelmintic drugs, such as praziquantel (PZQ), niclosamide, albendazole, and others [8, 20, 39, 40]. Therefore, the possible sources of infections could be minimized to the greatest extent possible, and the transmission of *T. solium* taeniasis/cysticercosis could be controlled.

The treatment of cysticercosis must be tailored to the location of the lesions, the stage of disease progression, and the host's immune response [41]. In most cases, antiparasitic drugs should be used to destroy live or degenerating cysticerci [9]. It has been reported that the therapeutic effects of albendazole and praziquantel treatments for cerebral cysticercosis are well understood, and the combination treatment using albendazole and praziquantel treatments can increase the therapeutic efficacy for cerebral cysticercosis [20]. However, due to their high toxicity, these drugs are used at concentrations that inhibit parasite growth and reproduction rather than killing them [42]. Thus, novel targets and compound classes with low toxicity and high efficacy at low doses are urgently needed for disease prevention, control, and intervention. Recently, a combination of pumpkin seeds and areca nut has been investigated against taeniasis, while praziquantel and albendazole are administrated concurrently against cysticercosis with promising efficacy and low side effects [3].

While adult worm infestations are largely asymptomatic, living in the intestine without causing harm, the larval stages, particularly cysts, can cause symptomatic pathologic symptoms, often leading to serious life-threatening conditions as they spread to other body parts such as the brain, muscles, or other organs including the liver. Depending on the patient's condition and cyst location, NCC is traditionally treated with chemotherapy or surgery. In severe cases, such as for NCC, surgery is required to lower intracranial pressure and resolve hydrocephalus [43, 44]. It is performed when cysts lodge in such areas of the brain that may cause CSF obstruction, resulting in hydrocephalus. Given the advances in minimally invasive techniques, minimally invasive neurosurgery can be successfully applied in cases of mild NCC (i.e., only a few cysts), especially in the case of a single cyst [45]. Surgery is the only option for ocular cysticercosis due to the risk of blindness from antiparasitic reactions, and asymptomatic subcutaneous or intramuscular cysticerci do not require treatment [3].

Surgical treatments are needed in some patients afflicted with cerebral cysticercosis with very high intracranial tension, but not all the cysticercus can be removed completely. Antiparasitic therapy cannot be substituted. Therefore, antiparasitic drugs are still required after surgery [20].

4. Ecological determinants

4.1 Intensive pig farming practice

In general, the pig industry in China has three breeding modes: backyard farm, specialized household farm, and large-scale commercial farm [23]. For thousands of years, small-scale farmers raised all sorts of pork in China. Prior to 1978, these so-called backyard farms, which raised fewer than five pigs per year along with crops and other livestock, produced at least 95 percent of the country's pork [46].

In 2007, backyard farmers accounted for approximately 27% of the national pork production though the smallholder share was much higher in some regions of China. For example, in Sichuan, the historic and current national leader in pork production was backyard farms, which contributed 70% of the entire pork in the province, compared to roughly 20% in Guangdong Province [23]. Feeding troughs, the human toilet, and the pigsty used to be always next to each other in those backyard farms, and pigs could easily consume human stool or contaminated food and water. Following China's Reform and Opening (which began in 1978), the structure of pig farming in China has changed extensively kicking off the trend toward large-scale commercial pig raising, which still continues today [46]. Production on these farms ranges from 500 to 50,000 pigs per year and is rapidly expanding. It is not unusual for a single company to produce 100,000 hogs in a single year [23]. In 1985, these farms accounted for only 2.5% of total pork production in the country, but by 2007, their share had increased to 22% [23]. In that situation, the human toilet and the pigsty were completely separated, and the pigs were not allowed to have direct access to consume human excreta or contaminated feeds and water. The specialized household farm (5–500 pigs per year) falls somewhere between the backyard farm and the large-scale commercial farm. In Sichuan, specialized households accounted for 25% of the total, while large-scale commercial farms contributed only 5% [23]. As farming practices have changed, it has become increasingly difficult for pigs to come into contact with human stool or contaminated feeds and water, and the transmission of *T. solium* would be cut off (**Figure 1**). As a result, if environmental reconstruction can create unfavorable conditions for these intermediate hosts, the *T. solium* transmission route could be disrupted, and the disease transmission could be minimized to a greater extent [21].

4.2 Human toilet revolution

Many pathogens can be found in human feces, including *T. solium* eggs, which can cause serious intestinal infections. The discharge of large amount of untreated feces sludge into the open environment endangers public health [47]. The human toilet revolution in extensively rural areas in China is a step-by-step campaign aimed at ensuring hygienic separation of human excreta from human contact, providing sanitary and comfortable space for users, preventing human excreta from polluting the environment, and realizing resource recycling [47].

The toilet revolution aims to increase the use of sanitary toilets, which definitely aids in disease prevention. During the ongoing toilet retrofitting campaign in rural areas, China has made significant progress. In China, the number of sanitary and innocuous-sanitary toilets has increased in the last decade, while significant regional diversification requires to be completed [48]. Sanitary toilet coverage in the rural areas has increased from 7.5% in 1993 to 78.5% in 2015, while harmless sanitary toilet coverage reached 57.5% by the end of 2015 [47]. The numbers have been increasing in most regions. Overall, the toilet revolution has made significant progress in improving sanitation infrastructure in rural China.

Currently, the concept of a toilet revolution is being enlarged and extended. Furthermore, it is not confined to the toilet, but to the entire sanitary system [47]. Consequently, pigs are getting very little opportunity to feed on human stool, and the transmission of *T. solium* between humans and pigs is being controlled.

5. Comprehensive prevention and control

5.1 From the porcine aspect

Comprehensive prevention and control encompasses chemotherapy for taeniid tapeworm carriers, cysticercosis patients and pigs in the community, as well as government initiatives for food safety laws, and meat inspections and regulations [16, 21]. Since 1970s, there have been surveillance and intervention measures for cysticercosis/taeniasis in endemic areas across the country through government health education and promotion programs [16]. Government and international funds have consistently supported the community-based investigations of cysticercosis and taeniasis in order to advance disease control efforts. In China, health education and promotion have proven to be effective in the control of *T. solium* taeniasis/cysticercosis [20, 21, 49].

Great efforts have been made in the last few decades to develop effective vaccines and novel chemotherapeutic agents for the purpose of immunizing pigs and preventing *T. solium* transmission between humans and pigs, and continue in progress [50]. In recent field trials, a vaccine for porcine cysticercosis (TSOL18) has been shown to be highly effective against naturally acquired infection with *T. solium* in pigs [6]. In the recent years, evidence of active elimination of *T. solium* transmission with the use of the porcine cysticercosis vaccine TSOL18 in combination with a single dose of oxfendazole treatment of pigs has been obtained from endemic areas of Cameroon [51]. Indeed, it has the potential to be an excellent tool in the fight against cysticercosis.

Mass treatment of taeniasis is a cost-effective control strategy in the endemic areas [52]. Oxfendazole has been shown to be an effective drug for curing pigs by eliminating the cysts and providing resistance to further infection. Educating farmers about the importance of resource management strategy to minimize such kind of infections will encourage them to invest more money on pig farms [53, 54].

Interventions focused on pigs will not only control the sources of taeniasis transmission but may also potentially ameliorate the economic value of the pigs. Preventing *T. solium* infection and treating cysticercosis in pigs obviously benefit the farmers financially and may lead to increased compliance with other control activities such as community-based screening, therapy, and health education [55].

5.2 From the human aspect

Poor hygiene, inadequate sanitation, the use of untreated or partially treated human waste in agriculture, improper food handling, lack of knowledge about the risk of infection while visiting endemic countries, and the consumption of raw or undercooked pork, particularly in/from regions where pigs are raised in poor conditions, all contribute to the spread of human taeniasis/cysticercosis [31, 33, 37, 38]. Moreover, person-to-person transmission should not be ignored [56, 57].

Enhancing sanitation and health education to improve sanitary and food hygiene practices, interventions consisting of human chemotherapy with better diagnostic tools for taeniasis, and porcine chemotherapy and immunization should all be included in the prevention and control of *Taenia* pp. infections and cysticercosis [58]. Co-infection of multiple helminthes and other parasites is very common in cysticercosis-endemic regions and countries. In order to develop effective integrated parasite control programs, health systems and services must consider the presence of various parasites [3]. According to the available data, implementation of a single approach to *T. solium* control is insufficient. Thus, an integrated approach is required to ensure long-term prevention and control.

5.3 From the ecological aspect

In the past few decades, significant efforts have been made and are still being realized to eliminate human cysticercosis. Among these efforts are health promotions, meat inspection, chemotherapy, and combined comprehensive measures, which no doubt are the primary control measures for the diseases [21]. However, some additional factors such as modification in pig farming practices and the development of modern toilets that could affect human and pig *T. solium* taeniasis/cysticercosis have also been identified. These preventive measures could significantly hinder the *T. solium* transmission route. Although these two factors were often mentioned in the previous articles [59–61], the fundamental significance for reducing human cysticercosis by minimizing disease transmission was not adequately addressed. The spread of *T. solium* taeniasis and cysticercosis is noticeably being gradually reduced along with the shift in pig farming practices from small-scale to large-scale intensive farms as well as the revolution made in the use of sanitary toilets by humans.

However, *T. solium* taeniasis and cysticercosis are still prevalent in some low-socioeconomic areas of China, particularly in rural communities in Sichuan, Yunnan, and Guangxi provinces, where pigs are reared in substandard management conditions, and the consumption of raw or undercooked pork is a traditional feeding habit [28, 31, 37, 58]. Therefore, in order to completely eliminate cysticercosis, promotion of health and education, meat inspection, and chemotherapy are warranted and must be continued in the days to come.

6. Conclusion

T. solium taeniasis/cysticercosis is an important food-borne zoonotic parasitic disease frequently transmitted worldwide between pigs and humans. Poor hygiene, inadequate sanitation, the use of untreated or partially treated human excreta in agriculture, improper food handling, lack of proper knowledge regarding the risk of infection while visiting the endemic countries, and the consumption of raw or under cooked pork (or viscera) particularly in/from regions where pigs are raised under poor conditions facilitate its spread.

Based on the epidemiological studies on taeniasis/cysticercosis in both humans and pigs, a number of factors have been identified to have contributed to decreasing trend of this disease in China over the last few decades. The promotion of health and education, meat inspection at slaughterhouses, and chemotherapies have significantly contributed to a marked decline in the prevalence of *T. solium* taeniasis/cysticercosis in China. Furthermore, the two most crucial measures, that is, the structural shift in pig farming from backyard to large-scale intensive farms, and the revolution made in the practice of using toilets to improve sanitary conditions created unfavorable conditions for the pigs (i.e. intermediate hosts) to acquire cysticercosis.

If any of the essential links to the source of infections are missing, infectious disease transmission can be disrupted, and no new infections could occur. The disease transmission nexus and its intensity are affected by natural and social factors. Therefore, to control and probably to eliminate cysticercosis, a One Health approach is required, which includes the provision of awareness and education, construction and proper usage of latrines, better farm management, treatment and/or vaccination of pigs, and timely treatment of infected human cases.

Author details

Junqiang Li[1,2] and Longxian Zhang[1,2]*

1 College of Veterinary Medicine, Henan Agricultural University, Zhengzhou, China

2 International Joint Research Laboratory for Zoonotic Diseases of Henan, Zhengzhou, China

*Address all correspondence to: zhanglx8999@henau.edu.cn

IntechOpen

© 2023 The Author(s). Licensee IntechOpen. This chapter is distributed under the terms of the Creative Commons Attribution License (http://creativecommons.org/licenses/by/3.0), which permits unrestricted use, distribution, and reproduction in any medium, provided the original work is properly cited.

References

[1] Saratsis A, Sotiraki S, Braae UC, et al. Epidemiology of *Taenia saginata* taeniosis/cysticercosis: A systematic review of the distribution in the Middle East and North Africa. Parasites & Vectors. 2019;**12**(1):113

[2] Trevisan C, Sotiraki S, Laranjo-González M, et al. Epidemiology of taeniosis/cysticercosis in Europe, a systematic review: Eastern Europe. Parasites & Vectors. 2018;**11**(1):569

[3] Qian MB, Xiao N, Li SZ, et al. Control of taeniasis and cysticercosis in China. Advances in Parasitology. 2020;**110**:289-317

[4] Assana E, Lightowlers MW, Zoli AP, et al. *Taenia solium* taeniosis/cysticercosis in Africa: Risk factors, epidemiology and prospects for control using vaccination. Veterinary Parasitology. 2013;**195**(1-2):14-23

[5] Pujari A, Bhaskaran K, Modaboyina S, et al. Cysticercosis in ophthalmology. Survey of Ophthalmology. 2022;**67**(2):544-569

[6] Lightowlers MW. Control of *Taenia solium* taeniasis/cysticercosis: Past practices and new possibilities. Parasitology. 2013;**140**(13):1566-1577

[7] Dixon MA, Winskill P, Harrison WE, et al. Global variation in force-of-infection trends for human *Taenia solium* taeniasis/cysticercosis. eLife. 2022;**11**:e76988

[8] Garcia HH, Gonzalez AE, Gilman RH. *Taenia solium* cysticercosis and its impact in neurological disease. Clinical Microbiology Reviews. 2020;**33**(3):e00085-e00019

[9] Garcia HH, Nash TE, del Brutto OH. Clinical symptoms, diagnosis, and treatment of neurocysticercosis. Lancet Neurology. 2014;**13**(12):1202-1215

[10] del Brutto OH, García HH. *Taenia solium* cysticercosis: New challenges for an old scourge. Pathog Glob Health. 2012;**106**(5):253

[11] O'Neal SE, Moyano LM, Ayvar V, et al. Ring-screening to control endemic transmission of *Taenia solium*. PLoS Neglected Tropical Diseases. 2014;**8**(9):e3125

[12] Gómez-Morales MA, Gárate T, Blocher J, et al. Present status of laboratory diagnosis of human taeniosis/cysticercosis in Europe. European Journal of Clinical Microbiology & Infectious Diseases. 2017;**36**(11):2029-2040

[13] Wandra T, Swastika K, Dharmawan NS, et al. The present situation and towards the prevention and control of neurocysticercosis on the tropical island, Bali, Indonesia. Parasit Vectors. 2015;**8**:148

[14] Dixon MA, Braae UC, Winskill P, et al. Strategies for tackling *Taenia solium* taeniosis/cysticercosis: A systematic review and comparison of transmission models, including an assessment of the wider Taeniidae family transmission models. PLoS Neglected Tropical Diseases. 2019;**13**(4):e0007301

[15] Hotez PJ, Bottazzi ME, Franco-Paredes C, et al. The neglected tropical diseases of Latin America and the Caribbean: A review of disease burden and distribution and a roadmap for control and elimination. PLoS Neglected Tropical Diseases. 2008;**2**(9):e300

[16] Wu HW, Ito A, Ai L, et al. Cysticercosis/taeniasis endemicity in Southeast Asia: Current status and control measures. Acta Tropica. 2017;**165**:121-132

[17] Flisser A. State of the art of *Taenia solium* as compared to *Taenia asiatica*. The Korean Journal of Parasitology. 2013;**51**(1):43-49

[18] Ito A, Wen H, Yamasaki H. Taeniasis/cysticercosis and echinococcosis in Asia. Asian Parasitology Series Monograph. 2005;**2**:1-334

[19] Carr KE. Water and Sewage in Ancient China. Quatr. Us Study Guides, June 7, 2017. Web. Feb. 18, 2019. Available from: https://quatr.us/china/water-sewage-ancient-china.htm.

[20] Wu W, Jia F, Wang W, et al. Antiparasitic treatment of cerebral cysticercosis: Lessons and experiences from China. Parasitology Research. 2013;**112**(8):2879-2890

[21] Wu W, Qian X, Huang Y, et al. A review of the control of clonorchiasis sinensis and *Taenia solium* taeniasis/cysticercosis in China. Parasitology Research. 2012;**111**(5):1879-1884

[22] Qian Y, Song K, Hu T, et al. Environmental status of livestock and poultry sectors in China under current transformation stage. Science of the Total Environment. 2018;**622-623**:702-709

[23] Schneider M. Feeding China's pigs: Implications for the environment, China's smallholder farmers and food security. Institute for Agriculture And Trade Policy. 2011. DOI: 10.13140/RG.2.1.5132.4967

[24] Xu LQ, Yu SH, Xu SM. Distribution and pathogenic impact of human parasites in China. In: Distribution &Pathogenic Impact of Human Parasites in China. Vol. 227-228. Beijing: People's Medical Publishing House; 1999. pp. 606-607

[25] Hotez PJ, Zheng F, Long-qi X, et al. Emerging and reemerging helminthiases and the public health of China. Emerging Infectious Diseases. 1997;**3**(3):303-310

[26] Coordinating Office of the National Survey on the Important Human Parasitic Diseases (CONSIHPD). A national survey on current status of the important parasitic disease in human population. The Chinese Journal of Parasitology and Parasitic Diseases. 2005;**23**(5):332-340 (In Chinese)

[27] Chen Y, Zhou C, Zhu H, et al. National survey on the current status of important human parasitic diseases in China in 2015. The Chinese Journal of Parasitology and Parasitic Diseases. 2020;**38**(1):5-16 (In Chinese)

[28] Li H, Zang X, Qian M, et al. Current status and research progress of cysticercosis. Chinese Journal of Schistosomiasis Control. 2018;**30**(1):99-103

[29] Li T, Openshaw JJ, Chen X, et al. High prevalence of *Taenia solium* taeniasis and cysticercosis in Tibetan schoolchildren in western Sichuan, China: A cross-sectional study. Lancet. 2017;**390**:S89

[30] Qian M, Chen Y, Zhu H, et al. The design and interpretation of sampling for the national survey on important parasitic diseases in 2014-2015 in China. The Chinese Journal of Parasitology and Parasitic Diseases. 2021;**39**(1):88-92 (In Chinese)

[31] Chung JY, Eom KS, Yang Y, et al. A seroepidemiological survey of *Taenia solium* cysticercosis in Nabo, Guangxi Zhuang autonomous region,

China. Korean Journal of Parasitology. 2005;**43**(4):135-139

[32] Openshaw JJ, Medina A, Felt SA, et al. Prevalence and risk factors for *Taenia solium* cysticercosis in school-aged children: A school based study in western Sichuan, People's Republic of China. PLoS Neglected Tropical Diseases. 2018;**12**(5):e0006465

[33] Steinmann P, Zhou XN, Li YL, et al. Helminth infections and risk factor analysis among residents in Eryuan county, Yunnan province, China. Acta Tropica. 2007;**104**(1):38-51

[34] Li H, Tang D. Comprehensive prevention and control measures of cysticercosis. Zhongguo Xumu Shouyi Wenzhai. 2016;**32**(009):134-134 (In Chinese)

[35] Geysen D, Kanobana K, Victor B, et al. Validation of meat inspection results for *Taenia saginata* cysticercosis by PCR-restriction fragment length polymorphism. Journal of Food Protection. 2007;**70**(1):236-240

[36] Chiesa F, Dalmasso A, Bellio A, et al. Development of a biomolecular assay for postmortem diagnosis of *Taenia saginata* Cysticercosis. Foodborne Pathogens and Disease. 2010;**7**:1171-1175

[37] Li T, Craig PS, Ito A, et al. Taeniasis/cysticercosis in a Tibetan population in Sichuan Province, China. Acta Tropica. 2006;**100**(3):223-231

[38] Yang YM, Li Z, Shi WX. Epidemiological investigation on the prevalence of *Taeina* around Erhai Lake of Dali, China. Journal of Pathology and Disease Biology. 2007;**109**:114 (In Chinese)

[39] Ahmad R, Khan T, Ahmad B, et al. Neurocysticercosis: A review on status in India, management, and current therapeutic interventions. Parasitology Research. 2017;**116**(1):21-33

[40] Ito A, Wandra T, Li T, et al. The present situation of human taeniases and cysticercosis in Asia. Recent Patents on Anti-Infective Drug Discovery. 2014;**9**(3):173-185

[41] Coyle CM. Neurocysticerosis: An individualized approach. Infectious Disease Clinics of North America. 2019;**33**:153-168

[42] Brunetti E, White AC Jr. Cestode infestations: Hydatid disease and cysticercosis. Infectious Disease Clinics of North America. 2012;**26**(2):421-435

[43] Bu XY, Liu M, Zhang JG, et al. Surgical treatment of brain cysticercosis patients with hydrocephalus. Henan Yi Xue Yan Jiu. 2009;**18**:193-195

[44] Yuan Z, Ren HJ, Wu XL, et al. Necessity of surgical intervention in the treatment of severe neurocysticercosis. Lanzhou Da Xue Xue Bao (Yi Xue Ban). 2005;**31**:30-32

[45] Zhang J, Zhang X, Cao WD, et al. Minimally invasive neurosurgery for neurocysticercosis. Di Si Jun Yi Da Xue Xue Bao. 2001;**22**:2191-2194 (In Chinese)

[46] Chen B, Yi B, Cheng F. History of the development of swine industry through the twenieth century in China. Journal of Xinyang Agricultural College. 2007;**17**(1):115-115 (In Chinese)

[47] Cheng S, Li Z, Uddin SMN, et al. Toilet revolution in China. Journal of Environmental Management. 2018;**216**:347-356

[48] Zhang S, Li Y, Zhang Y, et al. Does sanitation infrastructure in rural areas affect migrant workers' health?

Empirical evidence from China. Environmental Geochemistry and Health. 2020;**42**(2):625-646

[49] Cao W, van der Ploeg CP, Xu J, et al. Risk factors for human cysticercosis morbidity: A population-based case-control study. Epidemiology and Infection. 1997;**119**(2):231-235

[50] Wang L, Liang P, Wei Y, et al. *Taenia solium* insulin receptors: Promising candidates for cysticercosis treatment and prevention. Acta Tropica. 2020;**209**:105552

[51] Assana E, Kyngdon CT, Gauci CG, et al. Elimination of *Taenia solium* transmission to pigs in a field trial of the TSOL18 vaccine in Cameroon. International Journal for Parasitology. 2010;**40**(5):515-519

[52] Alexander A, John KR, Jayaraman T, et al. Economic implications of three strategies for the control of taeniasis. Tropical Medicine & International Health. 2011;**16**(11):1410-1416

[53] Kabululu ML, Ngowi HA, Mlangwa JED, et al. TSOL18 vaccine and oxfendazole for control of *Taenia solium* cysticercosis in pigs: A field trial in endemic areas of Tanzania. PLoS Neglected Tropical Diseases. 2020;**14**(10):e0008785

[54] Ngowi HA, Winkler AS, Braae UC, et al. *Taenia solium* taeniosis and cysticercosis literature in Tanzania provides research evidence justification for control: A systematic scoping review. PLoS One. 2019;**14**(6):e0217420

[55] O'Neal S, Noh J, Wilkins P, et al. *Taenia solium* tapeworm infection, Oregon, 2006-2009. Emerging Infectious Diseases. 2011;**17**(6):1030-1036

[56] Gonzalez AE, Lopez-Urbina T, Tsang B, et al. Transmission dynamics of *Taenia solium* and potential for pig-to-pig transmission. Parasitology International. 2006;**55**:S131-S135

[57] Rajshekhar V, Joshi DD, Doanh NQ, et al. *Taenia solium* taeniosis/cysticercosis in Asia: Epidemiology, impact and issues. Acta Tropica. 2003;**87**(1):53-60

[58] Gauci CG, Jayashi CM, Gonzalez AE, et al. Protection of pigs against *Taenia solium* cysticercosis by immunization with novel recombinant antigens. Vaccine. 2012;**30**(26):3824-3828

[59] Ito A, Li T, Wandra T, et al. Taeniasis and cysticercosis in Asia: A review with emphasis on molecular approaches and local lifestyles. Acta Tropica. 2019;**198**:105075

[60] Le TT, Vu-Thi N, Dang-Xuan S, et al. Seroprevalence and associated risk factors of trichinellosis and *T. Solium* cysticercosis in indigenous pigs in Hoa Binh Province, Vietnam. Tropical Medicine and Infectious Disease. 2022;**7**(4):57

[61] Rahantamalala A, Rakotoarison RL, Rakotomalala E, et al. Prevalence and factors associated with human *Taenia solium* taeniosis and cysticercosis in twelve remote villages of Ranomafana rainforest, Madagascar. PLoS Neglected Tropical Diseases. 2022;**16**(4):e0010265

Chapter 5

Neurocysticercosis: A Review on Global Neurological Disease

Km Deepika, Anshu Chaudhary, Bindu Sharma and Hridaya Shanker Singh

Abstract

The most prominent parasitic disease of the human central nervous system is neurocysticercosis, a neurologic parasite disease brought on by the engorged larva of the tapeworm *Taenia solium*. It is the most frequent cause of acquired epilepsy in endemic areas and a problem for the bulk of the developing world's public health systems. However, because of globalisation, neurocysticercosis cases are now also increasing in wealthy nations. With two intermediate hosts (i.e., pigs and humans) and one final host, neurocysticercosis has a complicated disease path, through faecal-oral contamination, one contracts it. Neurocysticercosis is the most significant CNS parasite that causes severe illness. Based on the location of the disease, it has historically been classified into active and inactive types. Radiologists must be aware of the differential diagnosis because of the wide variety of its imaging appearances. Imaging results are influenced by the number and distribution of parasites as well as any related consequences such as vascular involvement, an inflammatory response, and, in the case of ventricular forms, the degree of blockage. As a result, the diagnosis, treatment, and prognosis of neurocysticercosis vary widely depending on the type of infection.

Keywords: neurocysticercosis, neurologic, *Taenia solium*, neurocysticercosis treatment, neurocysticercosis diagnosis

1. Introduction

Initially recognised in ancient Greece as a pig disease, neurocysticercosis is the most prevalent helminthic disease of the human CNS. The majority of the developing world is affected by the disease, which thrives in environments with a warm climate, extreme deprivation, and widespread illiteracy. The disease is a health concern in metropolitan areas of developing countries because neurocysticercosis is a significant contributor [1–3]. In the industrialised world, the prevalence of neurocysticercosis has grown along with the number of immigrants coming from endemic countries. Latin American immigrants account for approximately 90% of neurocysticercosis patients in the United States and Europe [4–6]. However, neurocysticercosis has also been seen in people who have never travelled to a location where it is endemic. The majority of these people become ill after being exposed to an adult *T. solium* in their bowel [7]. The host's immunological response to the cysticerci pleomorphic lesions that parasites generate in the body is sporadic, and the condition is intriguing because it affects the CNS. Neurocysticercosis has sparked a great deal of interest due to medications. Here, we'll go over the key elements of this emphasis on the pathogenesis of parasitic diseases, and on current developments in diagnosis and treatment.

2. Etiopathogenesis

The life cycle of *T. solium* completes within two hosts (**Figure 1**). Pigs and humans can both act as intermediate hosts for the tapeworm metacestode stage called cysticercus larvae, but humans are the permanent host. During the typical cycle of transmission, the adult *Theridion solium* resides in the human small intestine, where it is affixed to the intestinal wall by its powerful suckers and hooks. The gravid proglottids, which are connected to the worm's distal end, are separated and passed with the faeces, release thousands of viable eggs into the environment. In places with inadequate faeces disposal, pork is fed with human faeces bearing *T. solium* eggs. The eggs shed their outer covers once they are within the pig's digestive tract, releasing oncospheres that go through the intestinal wall and into the circulation before being transported to the tissues, where they develop into cysticercus. Cysticerci are produced in the small intestine, after people consume tainted hog meat, where the action of digestive enzymes leads their scolices to evaginate and adhere to the intestinal wall.

Once the scolex is attached, the proglottids proliferate until they reach maturity 4 months after infection [9]. Humans can act as intermediate hosts for *T. solium* after eating its eggs. Under these circumstances, human cysticercosis can occur. Cysticercosis can be contracted from faeces by people who consume food contaminated with *T. solium* eggs or by those who already have the adult parasite in their intestines. Previous hypotheses that claimed that environmental contamination with *T. solium* eggs was the main cause of human contamination with the parasite have been disproved by recent epidemiological research that shows the clustering of cysticercosis patients near taeniasis patients. Human cysticercosis is considered to be an illness that primarily spreads from person to person, with infected pigs acting as the vehicle for the parasites [10].

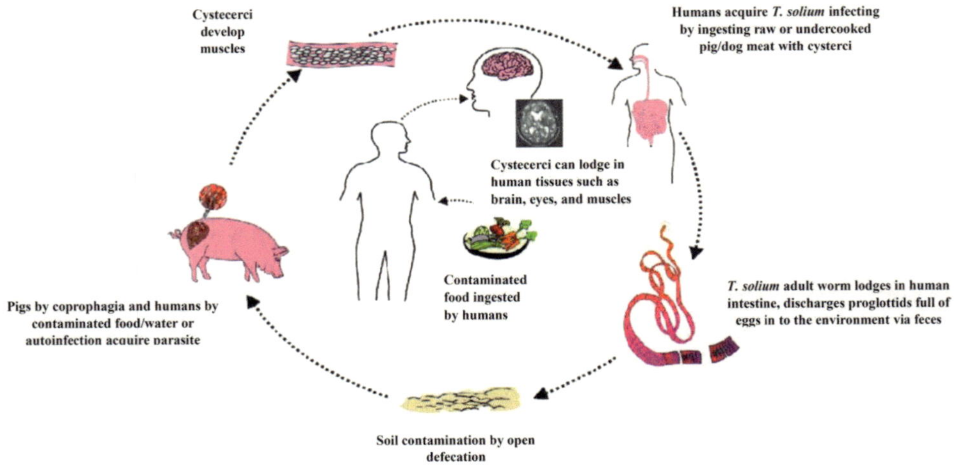

Figure 1.
Life cycle of Neurocysticercosis (Source: [8]).

The two main parts of cysticerci are the scolex and the vesicular wall [11]. After entering the central nervous system, cysticerci are in the vesicular (viable) stage, when the parasites have a transparent membrane, clear vesicular fluid, and a characteristically invaginated scolex. Cysticerci may last for years or undergo a degenerative process that causes them to turn into calcifications as a result of the host's immune response. The vesicular fluid becomes murky during the colloidal stage of cysticercal involution, and the scolex shows signs of hyaline degeneration. During the next stage, known as the granular stage, the cyst wall hardens and the scolex changes into mineralised granules. The cysticercus is no longer alive at this moment. Finally, the parasite remains are visible as a mineralised nodule [12]. The tissue around vesicular cysticerci does not experience considerable inflammation. In contrast, the parasite is typically wrapped in a collagen capsule, with a mononuclear inflammatory response surrounding colloidal cysticerci.

The surrounding brain parenchyma exhibits astrocyte gliosis, microglial proliferation, oedema, neuronal degenerative changes, and lymphocyte perivascular cuffing. When the parasites reach the granular and calcified phases, the oedema disappears; however, the astrocytic changes around the lesions may worsen. Epithelioid cells also begin to grow and assemble into multinucleated big cells at this time. Meningeal cysticerci often cause a strong inflammatory response in the subarachnoid space and aberrant thickening of the leptomeninges. This exudate contains collagen fibres, lymphocytes, multinucleated giant cells, eosinophils, and hyalinized parasite membranes [13]. Widespread inflammation may cause damage to cranial nerves, the optic chiasm, and small penetrating arteries that arise from the circle of Willis.

The latter might result in a blockage of the vessel's lumen, which would cause a cerebral infarction to form [14]. Ventricular cysticerci may potentially trigger an inflammatory response if they are linked to the choroid plexus or the ventricular wall.

While certain cysticerci antigens aid in the evasion of the immune system's defences against cysticerci, other cysticerci antigens, including (especially antigen B),

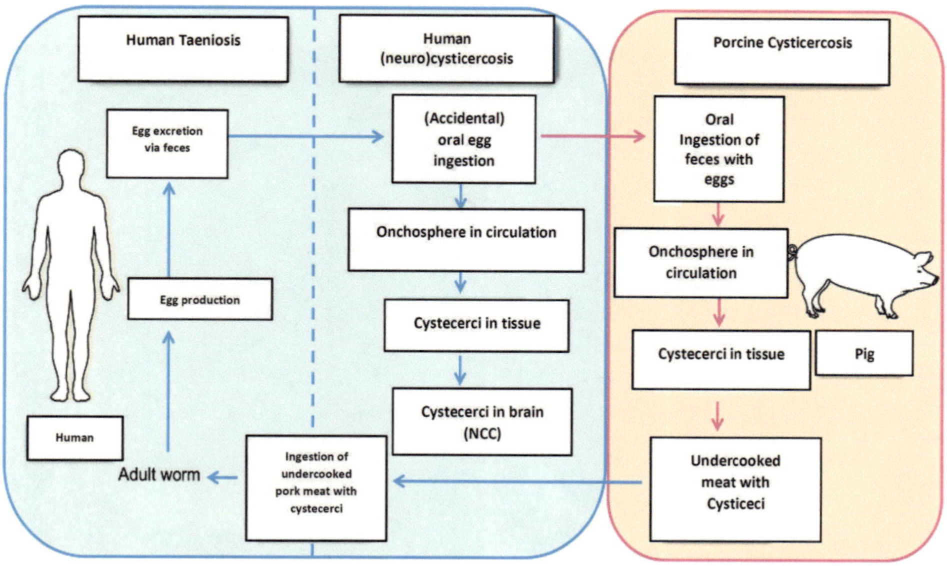

Figure 2.
Transmission of Neurocysticercosis. Source: https://journals.plos.org/plosntds/article/figures?id=10.1371/journal.pntd.0 008005

cause the production of particular antibodies that constitute the cornerstone of the cysticercosis immunological diagnosis [15]. Furthermore, it has been postulated that increased subpopulations of CD8 T-lymphocytes, poor lymphocyte proliferation, and aberrant cytokine concentrations in neurocysticercosis patients lead to cellular immunological dysfunction. According to the studies, immunodeficiency conditions and the growth of gliomas are associated with neurocysticercosis [16].

According to a notion, the immune system may find it challenging to detect malignancy in these circumstances due to the high levels of glial proliferation around the parasites and the inhibition of cellular immune responses, resulting in the malignant transformation of astrocytes (**Figure 2**) [17].

3. Clinical manifestations

Individual variability in the number and location of lesions within the CNS, as well as variations in the intensity of disease activity, accounts for the clinical pleomorphism of neurocysticercosis. The most frequent symptom of neurocysticercosis is seizures, which may be the only or major symptom in over 70% of individuals [18]. Patients with parenchymal neurocysticercosis experience seizures more frequently than those with subarachnoid or ventricular illnesses [19].

4. Diagnosis

Modern neuroimaging techniques have significantly improved our ability to diagnose neurocysticercosis. The quantity and topography of lesions as well as their stage of involution may be objectively determined using computed tomography and magnetic resonance (**Figure 3**) [21, 22]. On computed tomography and magnetic resonance, vesicular cysticerci show up as tiny, spherical cysts that are clearly

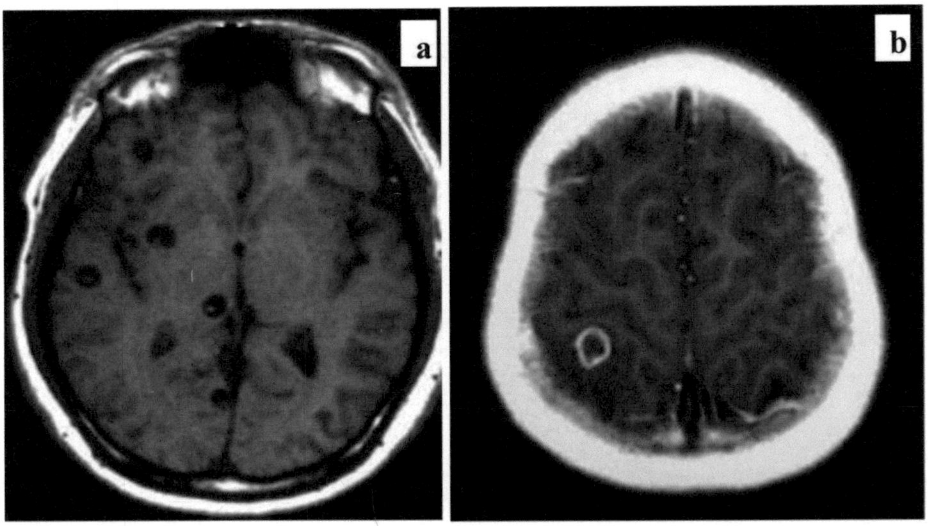

Figure 3.
Imaging with parenchymal brain cysticercosis: (a) viable cysts showing the scolex (b) colloidal cyst appearing as a ring-enhancing lesion [20].

Diagnostic criteria			
Absolute	**Major**	**Minor**	**Epidemiologic**
Histologic evidence of the parasite.	Neuroimaging investigations diagnosed the abnormalities	Neuroimaging studies	Household contact with suffering people
In neuroimaging studies, there is evidence of cystic lesions displaying the scolex.	Treatment of cerebral cystic lesions with albendazole or praziquantel.	Clinical symptoms of neurocysticercosis are seen.	where cysticercosis is endemic
The fundoscopic examination allows for the direct visualisation of subretinal parasites.	Anti cysticercal antibodies were detected in a positive serum immunoblot.	Presence of cysticercosis outside of the central nervous system.	

Table 1.
Table showing differential diagnostic criteria.

separated from the surrounding brain parenchyma. Physicians may now use a set of diagnostic criteria based on an unbiased assessment of clinical, radiological, immunological, and epidemiological data to help them identify individuals who may have neurocysticercosis (**Table 1**) [23]. Absolute, major, minor, and epidemiologic are the four types of criteria in this collection, which are ranked according to each diagnostic category's strengths.

The introduction of three-dimensional MRI sequences, such as Fast Imaging Employing Steady-State (FIESTA) and 3D constructive interferences steady state (3D CISS), has recently enhanced MRI sensitivity and specificity, particularly for subarachnoid and ventricular cysticerci [24–26]. Several approaches for detecting antigens and anti-cysticerci antibodies in CSF have been established. Although enzyme-linked immunosorbent assay (ELISA) and enzyme-linked immuno electro transfer blot assay (EITB) in CSF have good sensitivity and specificity, their complexity, length of execution, and cost are significant barriers to their use [27, 28]. *Taenia* antigens, which are more sensitive than eosinophils, can also be identified in CSF, particularly in clinically active kinds of NCC [28].

5. Treatment

There are four stages of neurocysticercosis completion (**Figure 4**). Based on which stage of neurocysticercosis is identified as are necessary for treatment, not every patient with neurocysticercosis is expected to respond favourably to a certain course of therapy. A well-informed treatment plan depends on accurately describing the illness in terms of the health of the cysts, the strength of the host's immune response to the worm, and the place and number of lesions [30]. Typically, treatment involves taking both symptomatic and cestocidal/cysticidal drugs. Additionally, surgery is used to treat certain individuals [31].

The prognosis for the majority of patients with neurocysticercosis has been considerably influenced by the widespread use of two potent cestocidal/cysticidal drugs (praziquantel and albendazole) [32]. Initial dosages of praziquantel were given for 15 days at a rate of 50 mg/kg/day (given every 8 hours) [33]. Then it was suggested that eliminating the parasites could only require three different doses of 25 to 30 mg/kg

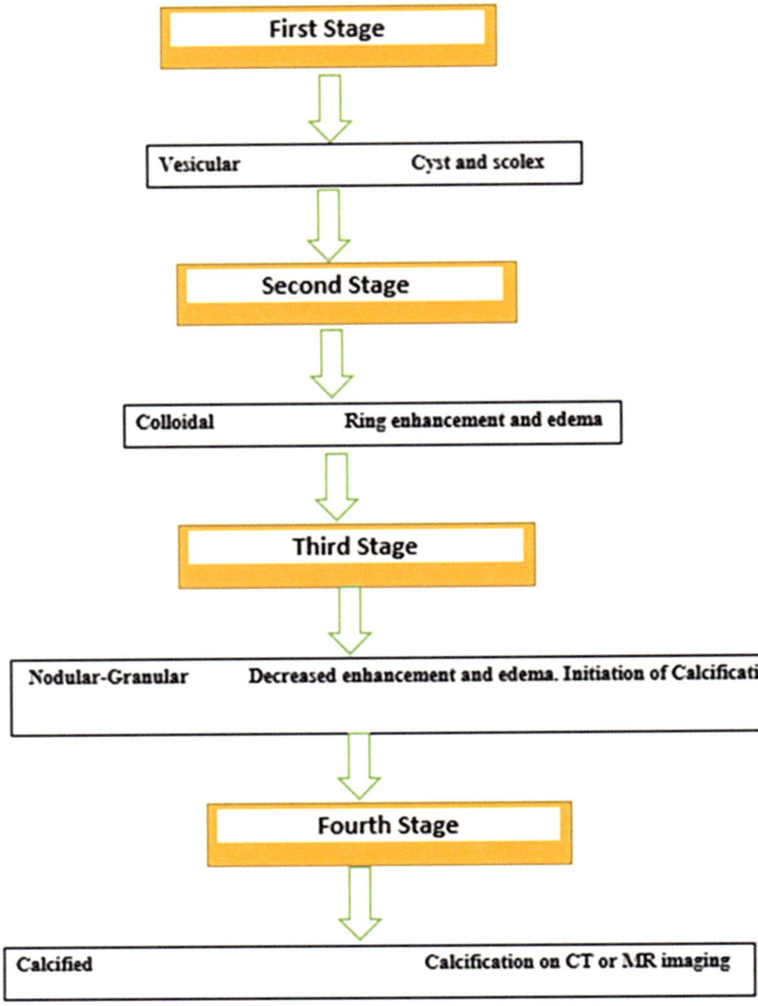

Figure 4.
Representing Stages of Neurocysticercosis [29].

given at intervals of 2 hours, exposing cysticerci to high drug concentrations sustained for up to 6 hours. It seems that patients with a single parenchymal brain cyst respond better to praziquantel's one-day therapy, but those with numerous cysts should utilise the 15-day trial, despite the early data with this unique regimen being encouraging.

Albendazole, the other cestocidal/cysticidal drug, was originally administered at dosages of 15 mg/kg/day for a month [34]. According to additional studies, if a patient just has a single brain cyst, the period of treatment might be shortened to just 1 week or perhaps just 3 days. In trials comparing the effectiveness of the two drugs, albendazole has outperformed by praziquantel. Another advantage of albendazole is that it removes ventricular and subarachnoid cysts. In some of these circumstances, especially in people with significant subarachnoid cysts, higher doses of albendazole (up to 30 mg/kg/day) or longer or even repeated courses may be necessary.

The use of cestocial/cysticidal medications has come under investigation due to the mild nature of some cases of neurocysticercosis, which has caused patient uncertainty and poor treatment choices. Cestocidal/Cysticidal medications are allegedly only effective at removing cysts; they have no impact on the clinical course of the disease. Recent studies, however, have shown that the majority of patients who use cestocidal/cysticidal drugs also see improvements in their clinical conditions. In a placebo-controlled study, albendazole was effective in treating viable parenchymal brain cysticerci [35–37].

Other well-conducted trials demonstrated that, in contrast to non-treatment, therapy improves the prognosis of individuals with colloidal parenchymal brain cysts. A recent meta-analysis of randomised controlled trials investigated the effects of cestocidal/cysticidal drugs on neuroimaging and clinical outcomes in patients with neurocysticercosis. According to that meta-analysis of published data, cestocidal/cysticidal drug therapy results in a lower risk of seizure recurrence in patients with colloidal cysticerci, a decrease in the frequency of generalised seizures in patients with vesicular cysticerci, and better resolution of both colloidal and vesicular cysticerci. Remember that not all neurocysticercosis patients should be treated with cestocidal/cysticidal drugs. These drugs may exacerbate the symptoms of intracranial hypertension found in cysticercotic encephalitis patients [36].

To avoid further therapy-related increases in intracranial pressure, cestocidal/cystocidal medicines should only be administered to patients with parenchymal brain cysts and hydrocephalus. Concurrent steroid administration is necessary to reduce the risk of a cerebral infarct. Individuals with ventricular cysts should refrain from taking cestocidal/cysticidal drugs. Last but not least, cestocidal/cysticidal drugs should not be administered to individuals who merely have calcifications because these lesions simply reveal parasites that are already dead. Patients with epilepsy brought on by neurocysticercosis often get seizure control after using just one first-line antiepileptic drug. According to some research, in order to effectively manage their seizures, patients with live intracranial cysts should first receive cestocidal/cysticidal medication before receiving antiepileptic medication [38].

It is unknown how long patients with neurocysticercosis should take antiepileptic medication. Prospective research found that up to 50% of patients with parenchymal brain cysticercosis who were successfully handled with cestocidal/cysticidal drugs later lost consciousness after quitting their antiepileptic drugs [39].

6. Control measures

T. solium transmission factors include inadequate faecal waste management practices, a lack of education, pig slaughter houses with no veterinary control, and the presence of wild pigs close to households, which are common causes of neurocysticercosis. The parasite condition could be fully eliminated. However, in order for eradication efforts to be effective, they must concentrate on complete control, such as with human adult tapeworm carriers, infected pigs, and environmental eggs. Inadequate focus on one of these targets might result in a subsequent increase in the prevalence of taeniasis and cysticercosis since these targets correspond to related phases in the life cycle of *T. solium* [36, 37].

7. Conclusion

The morbidity and mortality of the NCC are strongly impacted by accurate diagnosis together with appropriate symptomatic assessment, followed by a well-designed therapeutic intervention by the healthcare professional. Potential research avenues include the creation of novel cestocidal/cysticidal medications and drug delivery technologies for both the human and swine populations [8].

8. Future prospects

With an understanding of these immunological and genetic pathways, more modern drugs like tamoxifen and cutting-edge drug delivery techniques like lactic acid-conjugated solid lipid nanoparticles carrying albendazole and prednisolone will be created to successfully treat NCC. Preclinical animal studies on the pharmacokinetics, safety, and toxicity of oxfendazole for humans have yielded encouraging findings. For the management of swine cysticercosis, another promising area of study is the development of potent antiparasitic drugs, particularly in combination therapy, [40].

9. Preventive measures

There are many issues, including a lack of adequate epidemiological data on infection, control, and elimination. Suspected cases can be avoided through community health and education efforts, as well as a comprehensive healthcare approach involving [41–44].

- Pig vaccination and anthelmintic medication to prevent *T. solium* cysticercosis infection.
- Updated pig management procedures to keep pigs away from human excrement.
- Inspection and adequate cooking of pigs to limit the danger of human infection.
- Healthcare promoting hand cleanliness, food hygiene, sanitation, and pig management.

Acknowledgements

The authors are grateful for the facilities provided by the Department of Zoology, Chaudhary Charan Singh University, Meerut, India.

Conflict of interest

None

Author details

Km Deepika[1], Anshu Chaudhary[2*], Bindu Sharma[1] and Hridaya Shanker Singh[2,3]

1 Laboratory of Molecular Parasitology, Department of Zoology, Chaudhary Charan Singh University, Meerut, India

2 Molecular Taxonomy Laboratory, Department of Zoology, Chaudhary Charan Singh University, Meerut, India

3 Maa Shakumbhari University, India

*Address all correspondence to: anshuchaudhary81@gmail.com

IntechOpen

© 2023 The Author(s). Licensee IntechOpen. This chapter is distributed under the terms of the Creative Commons Attribution License (http://creativecommons.org/licenses/by/3.0), which permits unrestricted use, distribution, and reproduction in any medium, provided the original work is properly cited.

References

[1] Del Brutto OH, Santibanez R, Idrovo L, et al. Epilepsy and neurocysticercosis in Atahualpa: A door-to-door survey in rural coastal Ecuador. Epilepsia. 2005;**46**(4):583-587

[2] Medina MT, Duron RM, Martinez L. Prevalence, incidence, and etioloy of epilepsies in rural Honduras: The Salama study. Epilepsia. 2005;**46**:124-131

[3] Montano SM, Villaran MV, Ylquimiche L, et al. Neurocysticercosis: Association between seizures, serology, and brain CT in rural Peru. Neurology. 2005;**65**(2):229-234

[4] White AC Jr. Neurocysticercosis: Updates on epidemiology, pathogenesis, diagnosis, and management. Annual Review of Medicine. 2000;**51**:187-206

[5] Mas-Sesé G, Vives-Piñera I, Fernández-Barreiro A, et al. Estudio descriptivo de neurocisticercosis en un hospital terciario. Revista de Neurologia. 2008;**46**(4):194-196

[6] Serpa JA, Graviss EA, Kass JS, White AC. Neurocysticercosis in Houston, Texas: An update. Medicine. 2011;**90**(1):81-86

[7] Sorvillo F, Wilkins P, Shafir S, Eberhard M. Public health implications of cysticercosis acquired in the United States. Emerging Infectious Diseases. 2011;**17**(1):1-6

[8] Siddiqua T, Habeeb A. Neurocysticercosis. Saudi Journal of Kidney Diseases and Transplantation. 2020;**31**(254):2020. DOI: 10.4103/1319-2442.279948

[9] Del Brutto OH, Sotelo J, Roman G. Neurocysticercosis: A Clinical Handbook. Lisse, The Netherlands: Swets & Zeitlinger; 1988

[10] Gonzalez AE, Lopez-Urbina T, Tsang B, et al. Transmission dynamics of *Taenia solium* and potential for pig-to-pig transmission. Parasitology International. 2006;**55**:S131-S135

[11] Willms K. Morphology and biochemistry of the pork tapeworm, *Taenia solium*. Current Topics in Medicinal Chemistry. 2008;**8**(5):375-382

[12] Escobar A, Weidenheim KM. The pathology of neurocysticercosis. In: Singh G, Prabhakar S, editors. *Taenia solium* Cysticercosis. From Basic to Clinical Science. Oxon, UK: CAB International; 2002. pp. 289-305

[13] Pittella JEH. Neurocysticercosis. Brain Pathology. 1997;**7**(1):681-693

[14] Del Brutto OH. Stroke and vasculitis in patients with cysticercosis. In: Caplan LR, editor. Uncommon Causes of Stroke. New York, NY, USA: Cambridge University Press; 2008. pp. 53-58

[15] Flisser A, Correa D, Evans CAW. *Taenia solium* Cysticercosis. In: Singh G, Prabhakar S, editors. From Basic to Clinical Science. Oxon, UK: CAB International; 2002

[16] Del Brutto OH, Castillo PR, Mena IX, Freire AX. Neurocysticercosis among patients with cerebral gliomas. Archives of Neurology. 1997;**54**(9):1125-1128

[17] Del Brutto OH, Dolezal M, Castillo PR, García HH. Neurocysticercosis and oncogenesis. Archives of Medical Research. 2000;**31**(2):151-155

[18] Del Brutto OH, Santibañez R, Noboa CA, Aguirre R, Díaz E,

Alarcon TA. Epilepsy due to neurocysticercosis: Analysis of 203 patients. Neurology. 1992;**42**(2):389-392

[19] Garcia HH, Del Brutto OH. Neurocysticercosis: Updated concepts about an old disease. The Lancet Neurology. 2005;**4**(10):653-661

[20] Del Brutto OH. Neurocysticercosis: A review. The Scientific World Journal. 2012:159821. DOI: 10.1100/2012/159821

[21] García HH, Del Brutto OH. Imaging findings in neurocysticercosis. Acta Tropica. 2003;**87**(1):71-78

[22] Garcia HH, Del Brutto OH, Nash TE, White AC, Tsang VCW, Gilman RH. New concepts in the diagnosis and management of neurocysticercosis (*Taenia solium*). American Journal of Tropical Medicine and Hygiene. 2005;**72**(1):3-9

[23] Del Brutto OH, Rajshekhar V, White AC, et al. Proposed diagnostic criteria for neurocysticercosis. Neurology. 2001;**57**(2):177-183

[24] FEF M'AF, Machado LR, Lucato LT, Leite CC. The role of 3D volumetric MR sequences in diagnosing intraventricular neurocysticercosis: Preliminar results. Arquivos de Neuro-Psiquiatria. 2011;**69**(1):74-78. DOI: 10.1590/S0004-282X2011000100015

[25] Carrillo Mezo R, Lara García J, Arroyo M, Fleury A. Relevance of 3D magnetic resonance imaging sequences in diagnosing basal subarachnoid neurocysticercosis. Acta Tropica. 2015;**152**:60-65. DOI: 10.1016/j.actatropica.08.017.2015

[26] White AC Jr, Coyle CM, Rajshekhar V, Singh G, Hauser WA, Mohanty A, et al. Diagnosis and treatment of neurocysticercosis: 2017 Clinical practice guidelines by the Infectious Diseases Society of America (IDSA) and the American Society of Tropical Medicine and Hygiene (ASTMH). The American Journal of Tropical Medicine and Hygiene. 2018;**98**(4):945-966. DOI: 10.4269/ajtmh.18-88751

[27] Proaño-Narvaez JV, Meza-Lucas A, Mata-Ruiz O, García-Jerónimo RC, Correa D. Laboratory diagnosis of human neurocysticercosis: Double-blind comparison of enzyme-linked immunosorbent assay and electroimmunotransfer blot assay. Journal of Clinical Microbiology. 2002;**40**(6):2115-2118. DOI: 10.1128/JCM.40.6.2115-2118

[28] Gekeler F, Eichenlaub S, Mendoza EG, Sotelo J, Hoelscher M, Loscher T. Sensitivity and specificity of ELISA and immunoblot for diagnosing neurocysticercosis. European Journal of Clinical Microbiology & Infectious Diseases. 2002;**21**(3):227-229. DOI: 10.1007/s10096-002-0695-3

[29] Hanagandi PB, Gonçalves FG, do Amaral LLF, Chong JJR, Chankowsky J, Torres CI, et al. Multidisciplinary Approach to Tropical and Subtropical Infectious Diseases: Imaging with Pathologic Correlation. Neurographics. 2015;**5**(6):258-278. DOI: 10.3174/ng.6150133

[30] García HH, Evans CAW, Nash TE, et al. Current consensus guidelines for treatment of neurocysticercosis. Clinical Microbiology Reviews. 2002;**15**(4):747-756

[31] Nash TE, Singh G, White AC, et al. Treatment of neurocysticercosis: Current status and future research needs. Neurology. 2006;**67**(7):1120-1127

[32] Sotelo J, Diaz-Olavarrieta C. Neurocysticercosis: Changes after

25 years of medical therapy. Archives of Medical Research. 2010;**41**(1):62-63

[33] Sotelo J, Escobedo F, Rodriguez-Carbajal J, et al. Therapy of parenchymal brain cysticercosis with praziquantel. New England Journal of Medicine. 1984;**310**(16):1001-1007

[34] Escobedo F, Penagos P, Rodriguez J, Sotelo J. Albendazole therapy for neurocysticercosis. Archives of Internal Medicine. 1987;**147**(4):738-741

[35] Baranwal AK, Singhi PD, Khandelwal N, Singhi SC. Albendazole therapy in children with focal seizures and single small enhancing computerized tomographic lesions: A randomized, placebo-controlled, double blind trial. Pediatric Infectious Disease Journal. 1998;**17**(8):696-700

[36] Pawlowski ZS. Role of chemotherapy of taeniasis in prevention of neurocysticercosis. Parasitology International. 2006;**55**:S105-S109

[37] Codd EE, Ng HH, McFarlane C, et al. Preclinical studies on the pharmacokinetics, safety, and toxicology of oxfendazole: Toward first in human studies. International Journal of Toxicology. 2015;**34**:129-137

[38] Garcia HH, Pretell EJ, Gilman RH, et al. A trial of antiparasitic treatment to reduce the rate of seizures due to cerebral cysticercosis. New England Journal of Medicine. 2004;**350**(3):249-258

[39] Keilbach NM, De Aluja AS, Sarti-Gutierrez E. A programme to control taeniasis-cysticercosis (*T. solium*): Experiences in a Mexican village. Acta Leidensia. 1989;**57**(2):181-189

[40] Panic G, Duthaler U, Speich B, Keiser J. Repurposing drugs for the treatment and control of helminth infections. International Journal for Parasitology: Drugs and Drug Resistance. 2014;**4**:185-200

[41] Organização Mundial da Saúde. WHO Guidelines on Management of *Taenia solium* Neurocysticercosis. Geneva: World Health Organization; 2021

[42] Takayanagui OM, Castro e Silva AA, Santiago RC, Odashima NS, Terra VC, Takayanagui AMM. Compulsory notification of cysticercosis in Ribeirão Preto, SP, Brazil. Arquivos de Neuro-Psiquiatria. 1996;**54**(4):557-564. DOI: 10.1590/S0004-282X1996000400002

[43] Takayanagui OM, Febrônio LHP, Bergamini AMM, Okino MH, Silva AA, Santiago R, et al. Monitoring of lettuce crops of Ribeirão Preto, SP, Brazil. Revista da Sociedade Brasileira de Medicina Tropical. 2000;**33**(2):169-174. DOI: 10.1590/S0037-86822000000200002

[44] Takayanagui OM, Oliveira CD, Bergamini AMM, Capuano DM, Okino MH, Febrônio LH, et al. Monitoring of vegetables sold in Ribeirão Preto, SP, Brazil. Revista da Sociedade Brasileira de Medicina Tropical. 2001;**34**(1):37-41. DOI: 10.1590/S0037-86822001000100006

Chapter 6

Advances in the Diagnosis of Cysticercosis

Hassan Mohammad Tawfeeq

Abstract

Human cysticercosis is one of the most pathogenic and lethal diseases. It is caused by the accidental ingestion of *Taenia solium* eggs. All *Taenia* species lead to cysticercosis in animals; *T. solium* and *Torenia asiatica* are responsible for cysticercosis in pigs, while *T. saginata* causes bovine cysticercosis. Cysticercosis in humans is considered a neglected tropical disease. Diagnosing taeniasis—an infection with the adult parasite—poses challenges. The clinical manifestations of the disease are nonspecific, and no easy method is available to confirm the diagnosis. The diagnosis of cysticercosis is mainly based on imaging techniques, including computed tomography and magnetic resonance. These techniques are valuable and accurate but sometimes limited due to atypical images that are difficult to distinguish from neoplasms. Therefore, sensitive and specific methods, such as immunological tests and molecular methods, are essential to confirm clinical findings and differentiate cysticercosis from other diseases.

Keywords: *Taenia solium*, cysticercosis, neuroimaging, immunodiagnosis, molecular diagnosis

1. Introduction

Taeniasis and cysticercosis (T/C) are zoonotic infections caused by tapeworms of the genus *Taenia*. Humans are definitive hosts for three *Taenia* species that can cause human taeniasis: *Theridion solium*, *Theridion saginata*, and *Torenia asiatica* [1]. Cysticercosis refers to the tissue infection of the intermediate host: bovines for *T. saginata* and pigs for *T. solium* and *T. asiatica*—the first one is endemic to many developing regions, while the latter is restricted to some Asian countries [2]. Humans can get infected by ingesting raw or undercooked meat contaminated with cysticerci (larval cysts). However, humans can get infected with *T. solium* by consuming food or water contaminated with parasite eggs and act as dead-end intermediate hosts, developing cysticercosis. This infection often leads to neurocysticercosis (NCC), a major cause of epilepsy associated with considerable morbidity and mortality [3].

Neurocysticercosis is currently the most prevalent helminthic infection of the central nervous system (CNS). Although its prevalence is unknown, millions of people are likely infected with this parasite, and many eventually develop clinical symptoms. Most nations in Latin America, sub-Saharan Africa, and parts of Asia have endemic NCC. However, it is not typical in Northern Europe, the US, Canada, Australia, Japan, or New Zealand—except among immigrant communities [4].

IntechOpen

T. solium and *T. saginata* are flat, segmented, and hermaphrodite parasites measuring 2–10 m. Adult parasites are located in the small intestine. They comprise a head—or scolex—with a diameter of ~1 mm bearing four muscular suckers for fixation and some form of locomotion. Unlike *T. saginata*, *T. solium* has an armed rostellum bearing 22–36 hooks ordered in two rows. A thin neck measuring ~5–10 mm constitutes the portion with the most biokinetic activity; the entire body—or strobila—is formed from this part [5]. The adult *T. asiatica* worm measures 3.41 m in length and 9.5 mm in width and comprises 712 segments. The scolex of adult or larva *T. asiatica* has four suckers of 0.24–0.29 mm in diameter and a cuspidal rostellum with a maximal width of up to 0.81 mm. The maximum width of the *T. asiatica* scolex is 1.5 times smaller than that of *T. saginata* [6]. The strobila of *Taenia* species comprises 800–4000 proglottids—or segments—divided into immature, mature, and gravid segments. Immature segments are wider transversely than longitudinally, whereas mature segments are square, with primary sexual organs fully developed. Finally, gravid segments are rectangular, with the longest axis running lengthwise; most primary genital organs are atrophied, while the uterus is almost entirely branched and filled with oncospheres.

Oncospheres, or spherical eggs, are found in the uterus and range from 29 to 77 μm for *T. solium*, 39 to 50 μm in *T. saginata*, and 33.8 to 40 μm in *T. saginata*. The eggs of *Taenia* species cannot be distinguished by conventional light microscopy [7]. A cysticercus is an ovoid vesicle with a translucent membrane and a 5–15 mm diameter. It is filled with a colorless liquid and has an invaginated scolex. The larval stage is called *Cysticercus* spp., more appropriately called a "metacestode" of *Taenia* spp. The term "cysticercus racemosus" is frequently used to describe a wild-growing *T. solium* cysticercus in humans. This metacestode has a degenerative form and is found in the meninges and ventricular system of the brain. Cysticerci can persist in the brain for many years before patients experience symptoms; in some instances, they may never. Pleomorphic symptoms and signs are frequently brought on by the degradation of cysticerci and the accompanying host immunological response. Epileptic seizures, headaches, focal neurological impairments, and indicators of elevated intracranial pressure are the most typical symptoms. Neurological manifestations depend on the number—single or multiple—size, location (e.g., intraparenchymal or extraparenchymal), stage of the cysticerci—viable or calcified—and the host's immune response [8].

Researchers have been trying to develop diagnostic techniques to detect the presence of parasites within bodily tissues since the early 20th century. Counting white blood cells, specifically eosinophils, was an initial nonspecific test that raised the possibility of infections [9]. Serological tests for circulating antibodies (Abs) were created very quickly. Although unable to distinguish between active and dormant infections, antibody detection proved to be a better attempt at diagnosis, with greater predictive values than the earlier eosinophil counting [10]. The enzyme-linked immunosorbent test (ELISA), introduced in 1971, quickly gained popularity as the preferred method for detecting antibodies; it was the most sensitive method available at the time to process multiple samples simultaneously [11]. Computed Tomography (CT) and Magnetic Resonance Imaging (MRI), developed in 1977 and 1986, respectively, significantly improved the classification of NCC features [12]. These scans made it easier for clinicians to make definitive diagnoses based on the size, type, stage, and location of cysticerci in the patient's CNS. Neuroimaging is still the reference standard today.

2. Diagnosis

2.1 Clinical diagnosis

Although clinical history alone is insufficient for NCC diagnosis, healthcare professionals should become familiar with some of the nonspecific clinical manifestations, particularly in endemic regions [13]. NCC symptoms vary depending on the location, number, and size of the infecting worm(s), the duration of the infection, the evolutionary stage of the lesions, and the presence or absence of a cephalic budding cysticercus [14].

Patients with symptomatic NCC frequently appear with nonspecific signs that may not allow diagnosis. Seizures are the most prevalent manifestation, accounting for 70% of symptomatic cases, and can happen at any age [15]. Headaches, focal neurologic impairments, intracranial pressure, and cognitive deterioration are other clinical signs of the illness [13]. Focal neurological signs are uncommon and depend on where parasites are located in the nervous system or when a cysticercosis-related stroke occurs. Intracranial hypertension is mainly limited to people with hydrocephalus, cysticercotic encephalitis, and large subarachnoid or ventricular cysts [16].

Health professionals must gather epidemiological information about patients, such as travel history, birthplace, address, and awareness of past or present intestinal tapeworm infection in oneself or household members, in addition to clinical assessments [13, 17]. Based on clinical suspicion, neuroimaging and serological tests will be required to confirm or rule out a diagnosis. The target sites for cysticercosis detection are illustrated in **Figure 1**.

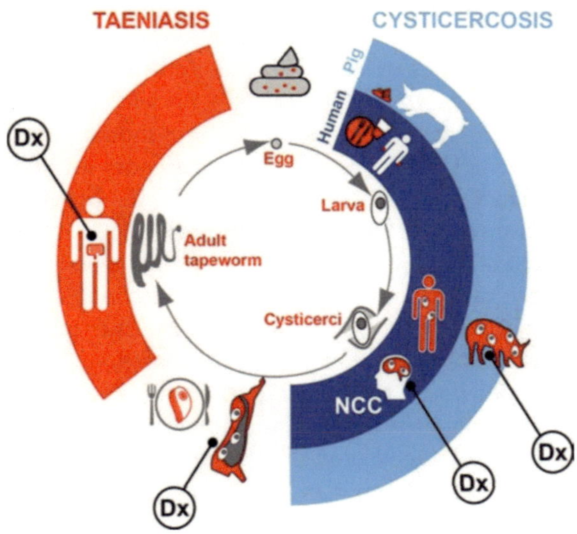

Figure 1.
Taeniasis/cysticercosis diagnostic tests (dx). Human: Adult tapeworm (taeniasis detection), larval cysts ([neuro] cysticercosis detection); pigs: Cysticerci in live pig or pork (cysticercosis detection).

2.2 Neuroimaging methods

Imaging techniques, such as CT and MRI, are essential because they can reveal the parasite's presence, number, location, size and stage, and the host's immune response, which manifests as diffuse or perilesional inflammation and blood-brain barrier dysfunction visible by focal contrast enhancement. Additionally, those techniques might indicate additional related diseases, such as hydrocephalus or a stroke [3, 18].

Both CT and MRI should be performed in patients with suspected NCC. MRI offers better imaging of tiny lesions, particularly those close to the skull and in the posterior fossa and provides more information on parenchymal inflammation or periventricular effusion in hydrocephalus [15, 19]. However, CT is considerably better at detecting calcifications and quantifying lesions and is more available in hospitals in endemic regions [20]. In addition to imaging studies, electroencephalography is useful in diagnosing NCC. It can provide a helpful map and the source of abnormal brain activity consistent with the regional distribution of lesions observed on CT scans [21, 22].

2.3 Laboratory diagnosis

2.3.1 Serologic diagnosis

Immunodiagnostic techniques are essential to support clinical results and help with diagnosis. Two immunological assays are available: antibody detection of past and current infections and antigen detection of recent infections. *T. solium* infection triggers the formation of a specific immunoglobulin G antibody that can be detected in serum and cerebrospinal fluid (CSF) [23].

Lentil lectin-purified glycoproteins are used in an enzyme-linked immunoelectrotransfer blot format in the serodiagnostic assay for cysticercosis and neurocysticercosis. They are approved by the World Health Organization and the Pan-American Health Organization [24]. Despite this assay's excellent sensitivity and specificity, antigen purification requires advanced techniques and specialized knowledge. It is not a quantitative assay and is challenging to apply in field research [25]. In addition, multiple types of antigens have been used for the immunodiagnosis of cysticercosis, including low molecular mass antigens, excretory/secretory antigens, crude soluble extract, total saline extract, antigen B, vesicular fluid, membrane and scolex extracts, somatic antigens, recombinant proteins, and synthetic peptides [26].

The major drawback of this approach is the possibility of false positives because antibodies do not always indicate an active infection with viable metacestodes but a resolved infection or exposure to the parasite [27]. Another disadvantage is the possibility of cross-reactivity with other parasitic diseases, such as the one caused by *Echinococcus granulosus*. However, cross-reactivity has also been reported with other diseases, including hymenolepiasis, fascioliasis, toxocariasis [28], toxoplasmosis, malaria, amoebiasis, cerebral tuberculosis [29], syphilis, and hepatitis [30].

There has been an increased interest in diagnosing NCC using new alternative antigenic sources because the presence or absence of antibodies cannot distinguish between different stages of the disease. A 2017 study by Nunes et al. used protein purification and gel filtration chromatography to identify potential heterologous antigens in a *T. solium* metacestode [31]. The study sought to discover specific polypeptides of interest and B cell epitopes for diagnosing NCC using gel filtration fractions and mass spectroscopy. Precursors of enolase and the calcium-binding protein calreticulin unique to the metacestode were discovered to have particular B cell epitopes indicative of NCC patients. Identifying these markers in serological samples is crucial and could be a reliable diagnostic tool for identifying NCC patients.

Detecting the specific circulating parasitic antigens can confirm the presence of viable parasites and overcome potential limitations. Several antigen detection techniques utilizing polyclonal or monoclonal antibodies have been studied. Two monoclonal antibody-based tests are standardized: B158/B60 Ag-ELISA and HP10. Antigen detection assays can also be used to monitor the efficacy of anthelminthic drugs and differentiate between viable parasites and locate them in the central nervous system [32]. A 2020 study by Kabululu et al. observed that the B158/B60 monoclonal-based sandwich enzyme-linked immunosorbent assay (Ag-ELISA) was more reliable in ruling out *T. solium* cysticercosis in pigs [33].

3. Histological study of the parasite from biopsy

Visualization of histopathological characteristics of cysticerci in biopsy material, including the spinal canal, the rostellum with its four suckers, and the double crown of hooks, can confirm NCC diagnosis. In many subarachnoid cysts, the scolex cannot be identified, but the typical three-layered membrane wall often allows the correct identification of the parasite. However, a problem arises when biopsy material comes from calcified or granular cysticerci since the scolex and membranes may not be present in these involution stages of the parasite. In such cases, the presence of the calcareous corpuscles may help identify the lesion's parasitic (cestode) nature [13].

3.1 Molecular techniques

PCR has been used for the amplification of DNA sequences. Since its creation by Mullis in 1983, PCR has developed into a crucial diagnostic tool. Several molecular assays have been described for the detection and differentiation of parasites, including *Taenia* species, using genomic or mitochondrial DNA: multiplex-PCR, nested PCR, quantitative real-time PCR, PCR-Restriction Fragment Length Polymorphism, a base excision sequence scanning thymine-base method (Yamasaki et al., 2002) and random amplified polymorphic DNA (RAPD) [34–38].

The most significant contribution of molecular methods has been in the genotyping of the genus *Taenia*, which has served to determine the phylogeny and taxonomy of the species and to understand the level of genetic diversity within the genus [38]. Another essential contribution of molecular biology was the identification and production of antigenic molecules used as candidates for vaccines or serological tests. Direct use of molecular techniques for NCC diagnosis was first reported in 2006. It identified *T. solium* DNA in the CSF of 29 out of 30 consecutive patients by PCR with primers against *pTsol9*, specific to *T. solium* [39, 40]. Another study found parasite DNA in human CSF, using primers against *HDP2*, based on a noncoding sequence of *T. saginata*, which cross-reacts with *T. solium*. The study also reported different sensitivities depending on the NCC type (10/14 for extraparenchymal NCC cases compared to 4/24 for intraparenchymal, degenerating NCC cases) [41].

MicroRNAs (miRNA) have recently been investigated as potential biomarkers. They are single-stranded, short, noncoding, endogenous RNAs with a role in post-transcriptional gene regulation. Although miRNAs have been linked to many parasites, little is known regarding *T. solium*. Possibly, during chronic infection, *T.*

solium manipulates the host's mRNA with miRNA to control the host-parasite interaction. Although these miRNAs have never been employed as biomarkers for infection diagnosis, they are increasingly recognized as novel disease regulators. To help with disease diagnosis and treatment, more investigation into the host-parasite interaction and miRNA is necessary [42].

Finally, neurocysticercosis remains a significant public health concern and financial burden in endemic areas. Numerous neurological symptoms caused by this parasite require expensive diagnostic methods. Despite efforts to create diagnostic techniques, serological analyses combined with neuroimaging currently serve as the primary diagnostic method. Neuroimaging is pricey and cannot detect isolated cysts or extraparenchymal infections. Additionally, the ideal serological biomarker remains elusive. Creating novel, trustworthy, and reasonably priced diagnostic techniques is crucial for the therapeutic management of this underappreciated tropical disease and for determining the actual global health burden it poses.

Author details

Hassan Mohammad Tawfeeq[1,2]

1 Nursing Department, Kalar Technical College, Sulaimani Polytechnic University, Kalar, Kurdistan Region, Iraq

2 Garmian Polytechnic University, Kalar, Kurdistan Region, Iraq

*Address all correspondence to: hassan.tawfeeq@spu.edu.iq

IntechOpen

© 2023 The Author(s). Licensee IntechOpen. This chapter is distributed under the terms of the Creative Commons Attribution License (http://creativecommons.org/licenses/by/3.0), which permits unrestricted use, distribution, and reproduction in any medium, provided the original work is properly cited.

References

[1] Flisser A. State of the art of Taenia solium as compared to Taenia asiatica. The Korean Journal of Parasitology. 2013;**51**:43-49

[2] Michelet L, Dauga C. Molecular evidence of host influences on the evolution and spread of human tapeworms. BRV Biological Reviews. 2012;**87**(3):731-741

[3] García HH, Del Brutto OH. Imaging findings in neurocysticercosis. Acta Tropica. 2003;**87**(1):71-78. DOI: 10.1016/s0001-706x(03)00057-3

[4] Del Brutto OH. Human Neurocysticercosis: An overview. Pathogens. 2022;**11**(10):1212. DOI: 10.3390/pathogens11101212

[5] Naquira C. *Taenia* solium: biological cycle and characteristics. In: Garcia HH, Martinez S, editors. Taenia solium Taeniasis, Cysticercosis. Lima: Editorial Universo; 1999. p. 346

[6] Eom KS. What is Asian Taenia? Parasitology International. 2006;**55**(Suppl):137-141

[7] Eom KS, Rim H. Morphologic descriptions of Taenia asiatica sp. n. The Korean Journal of Parasitology. 1993;**31**:1-6

[8] Abraham A, Schmidt V, Kaminski M, Stelzle D, De Meijere R, Bustos J, et al. Epidemiology and surveillance of human (neuro) cysticercosis in Europe: Is enhanced surveillance required? Tropical Medicine & International Health. 2020;**25**(5):566-578

[9] Waterhouse R. Cysticercus cellulosae in the central nervous system: With an account of two cases. QJM: An International Journal of Medicine. 1913;**6**(4):469-485

[10] Garcia HH, Gilman RH, Catacora M, Verastegui M, Gonzalez AE, Tsang VC. Serologic evolution of neurocysticercosis patients after antiparasitic therapy. Cysticercosis working Group in Peru. The Journal of Infectious Diseases. 1997;**175**(2):486-489

[11] Engvall E, Perlmann P. Enzyme-linked immunosorbent assay (ELISA). Quantitative assay of immunoglobulin G. Immunochemistry. 1971;**8**(9):871-874

[12] Chavarria A, Fleury A, Garcia E, Marquez C, Fragoso G, Sciutto E. Relationship between the clinical heterogeneity of neurocysticercosis and the immuneinflammatory profiles. Clinical Immunology. 2005;**116**(3):271-278

[13] Del Brutto OH, Nash TE, White AC Jr, Rajshekhar V, Wilkins PP, Singh G, et al. Revised diagnostic criteria for neurocysticercosis. Journal of the Neurological Sciences. 2017;**372**:202-210

[14] Garcia HH. Neurocysticercosis. Neurologic Clinics. 2018;**36**(4):851-864. DOI: 10.1016/j.ncl.2018.07.003

[15] Del Brutto OH, Santibañez R, Noboa CA, Aguirre R, Díaz E, Alarcón TA. Epilepsy due to neurocysticercosis: Analysis of 203 patients. Neurology. 1992;**42**(2):389-392

[16] Del Brutto OH, Del Brutto VJ. Calcified neurocysticercosis among patients with primary headache. Cephalalgia: An International Journal of Headache. 2012;**32**(3):250-254. DOI: 10.1177/0333102411433043

[17] Del Brutto OH. Diagnostic criteria for neurocysticercosis, revisited. Pathogens

and Global Health. 2012;**106**(5):299-304. DOI: 10.1179/2047773212Y.000000002

[18] Dumas JL, Visy JM, Belin C, Gaston A, Goldlust D, Dumas M. Parenchymal neurocysticercosis: Follow-up and staging by MRI. Neuroradiology. 1997;**39**(1): 12-18. DOI: 10.1007/s002340050358

[19] Carrillo Mezo R, Lara García J, Arroyo M, Fleury A. Relevance of 3D magnetic resonance imaging sequences in diagnosing basal subarachnoid neurocysticercosis. Acta Tropica. 2015;**152**:60-65. DOI: 10.1016/j.actatropica.2015.08.017

[20] Nash TE, Del Brutto OH, Butman JA, Corona T, Delgado-Escueta A, Duron RM, et al. Calcific neurocysticercosis and epileptogenesis. Neurology. 2004;**62**(11):1934-1938. DOI: 10.1212/01.wnl.0000129481.12067.06

[21] Sharma S, Modi M, Lal V, Prabhakar S, Bhardwaj A, Sehgal R. Reversible dementia as a presenting manifestation of racemose neurocysticercosis. Annals of Indian Academy of Neurology. 2013;**16**(1):88-90. DOI: 10.4103/0972-2327.107706

[22] Singh AK, Garg RK, Rizvi I, Malhotra HS, Kumar N, Gupta RK. Clinical and neuroimaging predictors of seizure recurrence in solitary calcified neurocysticercosis: A prospective observational study. Epilepsy Research. 2017;**137**:78-83. DOI: 10.1016/j.eplepsyres.2017.09.010

[23] Raoul F, Li T, Sako Y, Chen X, Long C, Yanagida T, et al. Advances in diagnosis and spatial analysis of cysticercosis and taeniasis. Parasitology. 2013;**140**(13):1578-1588. DOI: 10.1017/S0031182013001303

[24] Pan American Health Organization. PAHO/WHO Informal Consultation on the Taeniasis/Cysticercosis Complex. Brasilia, Brazil: Pan American Health Organization; 1995

[25] Lee YM, Handali S, Hancock K, Pattabhi S, Kovalenko VA, Levin A, et al. Serologic diagnosis of human Taenia solium cysticercosis by using recombinant and synthetic antigens in QuickELISA™. The American Journal of Tropical Medicine and Hygiene. 2011;**84**(4):587-593. DOI: 10.4269/ajtmh.2011.10-0079

[26] Esquivel-Velázquez M, Ostoa-Saloma P, Morales-Montor J, Hernández-Bello R, Larralde C. Immunodiagnosis of neurocysticercosis: Ways to focus on the challenge. Journal of Biomedicine and Biotechnology. 2011;**2011**:516042. DOI: 10.1155/2011/516042

[27] Garcia HH, Gonzalez AE, Gilman RH, Palacios LG, Jimenez I, Rodriguez S, et al. Transient antibody response in Taenia solium infection in field conditions-a major contributor to high seroprevalence. The American Journal of Tropical Medicine and Hygiene. 2001;**65**(1):31-32

[28] Dekumyoy P, Waikagul J, Vanijanonta S, Thairungroj M, Nakao M, Sako Y, et al. Cysticercosis: IgG-ELISA evaluations of peak1 antigen and< 30 kDa antigen of delipidized extract of Taenia solium metacestodes. Southeast Asian Journal of Tropical Medicine and Public Health. 2004;**35**:1-9

[29] Mandal J, Singhi PD, Khandelwal N, Malla N. Evaluation of lower molecular mass (20-24 kDa) Taenia solium cysticercus antigen fraction by ELISA and dot blot for the serodiagnosis of neurocysticercosis in children. Parasitology Research. 2008;**102**(5):1097-1101

[30] Arruda GC, Da Silva ADT, Quagliato EMAB, Maretti MA, Rossi CL.

Evaluation of Taenia solium and Taenia crassiceps cysticercal antigens for the serodiagnosis of neurocysticercosis. Tropical Medicine & International Health. 2005;**10**(10):1005-1012

[31] Nunes D, Gonzaga H, Ribeiro V, Cunha-Júnior J, Costa-Cruz J. Usefulness of gel filtration fraction as potential biomarker for neurocysticercosis in serum: Towards a new diagnostic tool. Parasitology. 2017;**144**(4):426-435

[32] Gadea NA, Matamoros G, Rueda MM. Recent advances in the diagnosis of Neurocysticercosis. Current Treatment Options in Infectious Diseases. 2018;**10**:410-420. DOI: 10.1007/s40506-018-0173-9

[33] Kabululu ML, Johansen MV, Mlangwa JED, et al. Performance of Ag-ELISA in the diagnosis of *Taenia solium* cysticercosis in naturally infected pigs in Tanzania. Parasites Vectors. 2020;**13**:534. DOI: 10.1186/s13071-020-04416-4

[34] Tawfeeq HM, Ali SA. Highly sensitive nested polymerase chain reaction to improve the detection of *Leishmania* species in clinical specimens. Journal of Parasitic Diseases. 2022;**46**(3):754-763. DOI: 10.1007/s12639-022-01491-5. Epub 2022 May 13. PMID: 36091274; PMCID: PMC9458810

[35] Tawfeeq HM, Ali SA. Molecular-based assay for genotyping Leishmania spp. from clinically suspected cutaneous leishmaniasis lesions in the Garmian area, Kurdistan region of Iraq. Parasite Epidemiology and Control. 2022;**17**:e00240

[36] Yamasaki H, Nakao M, Sako Y, Nakaya K, Sato MO, Mamuti W, et al. DNA differential diagnosis of human Taeniid Cestodes by base excision sequence scanning Thymine-Base reader analysis with mitochondrial genes. Journal of Clinical Microbiology. 2002;**40**:3818-3821

[37] Vega R, Pinero D, Ramanankandrasana B, Dumas M, Bouteille B, Fleury A, et al. Population genetic structure of Taenia solium from Madagascar and Mexico: Implications for clinical profile diversity and immunological technology. International Journal for Parasitology. 2003;**33**:1479-1485

[38] Nunes CM, Lima LGF, Manoel CS, Pereira RN, Nakano MM, Garcia JF. Taenia saginata: Polymerase chain reaction for taeniasis diagnosis in human fecal samples. Experimental Parasitology. 2003;**104**:67-69

[39] McManus DP. Molecular discrimination of taeniid cestodes. Parasitology International. 2006;**55**:S31-S37

[40] Almeida CR, Ojopi EP, Nunes CM, Machado LR, Takayanagui OM, Livramento JA, et al. Taenia solium DNA is present in the cerebrospinal fluid of neurocysticercosis patients and can be used for diagnosis. European Archives of Psychiatry and Clinical Neuroscience. 2006;**256**(5):307-310

[41] Hernández M, Gonzalez LM, Fleury A, Saenz B, Parkhouse RME, Harrison LJS, et al. Neurocysticercosis: Detection of Taenia solium DNA in human cerebrospinal fluid using a semi-nested PCR based on HDP2. Annals of Tropical Medicine & Parasitology. 2008;**102**(4):317-323

[42] Gutierrez-Loli R, Orrego MA, Sevillano-Quispe OG, Herrera-Arrasco L, Guerra-Giraldez C. MicroRNAs in *Taenia solium* neurocysticercosis: Insights as promising agents in host-parasite interaction and their potential as biomarkers. Frontiers in Microbiology. 2017;**8**:1905

Chapter 7

Neurocysticercosis: An Overview of Pathology and Pathogenesis

Güngör Çağdaş Dinçel, Saeed El-Ashram, Luís Manuel Madeira de Carvalho, Danielle Graham, Inkar A. Castellanos-Huerta, Victor M. Petrone-Garcia, Guillermo Tellez-Isaias, Beniamino T. Cenci-Goga and Luca Grispoldi

Abstract

Neurocysticercosis (NCC), a subtle parasite infection of the central nervous system, is a powerful example of the complex interaction between human behavior, zoonotic transmission, and neurological illness development. Given the disease's worldwide prevalence and potentially fatal neurological consequences, research into NCC is critical for advancing knowledge, creating effective diagnostic tools and treatment options, and adopting preventative measures to lessen the disease's impact. Cysticerci causes an immunological response in the CNS, resulting in inflammation and immune cell recruitment. The existence of intraventricular cysts, cysts in the cerebral aqueduct or fourth ventricle, and the degree of inflammation and scarring induced by the infection are all risk factors for the development of hydrocephalus. This book chapter provides an in-depth exploration of the pathology and pathogenesis of NCC, discussing the life cycle of the *Taenia solium* parasite, its invasion of the central nervous system, and the formation of cysticerci, as well as the diagnostic challenges and imaging findings, clinical manifestations, and potential neurological complications associated with NCC, serving as a valuable resource for medical professionals, researchers, and policymakers.

Keywords: neuroimmunopathology, neurocysticercosis, zoonotic transmission, neuropathology, *Taenia solium*

1. Introduction

Neurocysticercosis (NCC), an insidious parasitic infection of the central nervous system, is a compelling testament to the intricate interplay between human behavior, zoonotic transmission, and neurological disorder pathogenesis. Caused by the larval stage of the pork tapeworm, *Taenia solium*, NCC represents a significant global health burden, particularly in regions plagued by inadequate sanitation and poor hygiene practices. As a leading cause of acquired epilepsy worldwide, this enigmatic condition transcends geographical boundaries and socio-economic disparities, leaving a trail of neuroinflammatory cascades, structural aberrations, and clinical manifestations [1, 2]. Unraveling the complex neuropathological intricacies of NCC holds the key to understanding its multifaceted impact on the human brain, ultimately guiding the pursuit of effective diagnostic modalities, therapeutic interventions, and preventive strategies [1, 3, 4]. Through an amalgamation of meticulous clinical observation, cutting-edge neuroimaging techniques, and the unraveling of host-parasite interactions, the neuropathological landscape of NCC gradually unveils its enigmatic nature, beckoning the relentless quest for knowledge in the realm of neurology and parasitology [1, 3, 4].

NCC is a complex parasitic infection that elicits diverse neuropathological changes within the central nervous system. The development of neuropathology in NCC follows a progressive course characterized by distinct stages. In the early vesicular stage, the cysticerci, comprising fluid-filled bladders housing the tapeworm larvae, exhibit a translucent membrane and contain a scolex with hooklets [5, 6]. As the infection progresses to the colloidal stage, degenerative changes occur, leading to a granulomatous reaction. This granuloma, composed of a necrotic core, edema, fibrous capsule, and inflammatory cells, contributes to the clinical manifestations commonly associated with NCC, such as seizures, headaches, and focal neurological deficits [6, 7]. Over time, some cysticerci may undergo calcification, resulting in the calcified stage where the parasites become inert, and the host response aims to contain the infection. Developing these neuropathological features in NCC underscores the dynamic interplay between the parasite, the host immune response, and the structural alterations within the central nervous system. Therefore, the evaluation and examination of neuropathological findings are very important [5–7].

NCC is paramount in infectious diseases and neurology due to its significant impact on public health and its potential to cause severe neurological complications. This parasitic infection, caused by the larval stage of the pork tapeworm, *T. solium*, primarily affects the central nervous system (CNS). NCC is recognized as a leading cause of acquired epilepsy worldwide, particularly in regions where the parasite is endemic. It substantially burdens affected individuals, their families, and healthcare systems. Moreover, NCC can lead to various neurological manifestations, including seizures, hydrocephalus, focal neurological deficits, cognitive impairments, and even life-threatening complications [8, 9]. The complex interplay between the immune response, parasite-host interactions, and the localization of cysticerci within the CNS contributes to the diverse clinical presentations and challenges in diagnosis and treatment. Given its global prevalence and potential for devastating neurological sequelae, the study of NCC is essential for improving understanding, developing effective diagnostic tools and treatment strategies, and implementing preventive measures to mitigate the impact of this disease (**Figure 1**) [8, 9].

The proposed book chapter on NCC is necessary and of utmost importance in the medical and scientific community. NCC, caused by the larval stage of the pork tapeworm, *T. solium*, is a neglected tropical disease with a significant global impact on public health. Despite its prevalence and the severe neurological complications it can induce, there is a notable scarcity of comprehensive literature that systematically addresses various aspects of the disease. This chapter aims to fill this critical knowledge gap by providing a comprehensive and up-to-date synthesis of the current understanding of NCC. It will cover diverse topics, including the parasite's life cycle, epidemiology, clinical manifestations, diagnostic methods, treatment options, and preventive strategies. By consolidating evidence-based information and the latest research findings, the chapter will be an essential reference for medical practitioners, researchers, and policymakers. Moreover, the book chapter will raise awareness about this often overlooked disease,

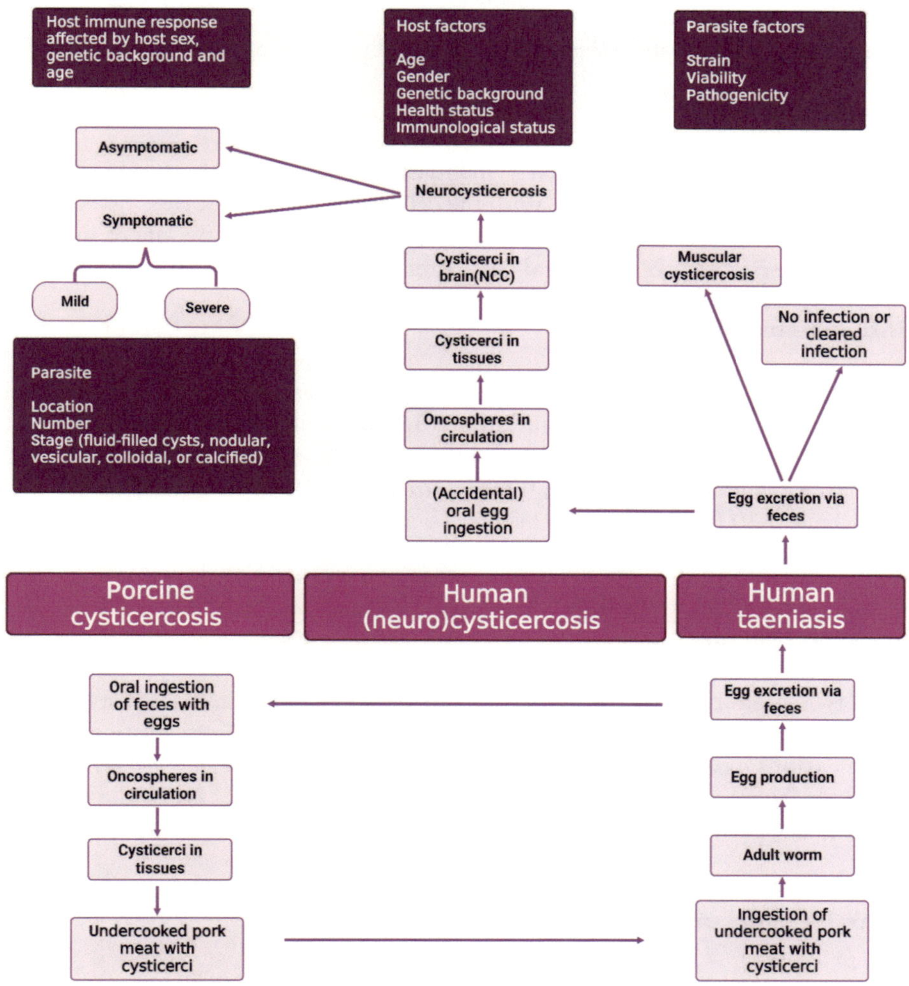

Figure 1.
T. solium infection depicting the stages of human and porcine cysticercosis, including NCC factors.

fostering international collaborations and research efforts to improve its diagnosis, management, and prevention. Ultimately, the chapter's significance lies in its potential to enhance the quality of patient care, contribute to scientific advancements, and alleviate the burden of NCC on affected communities worldwide.

2. Inflammatory response in neurocysticercosis

Cysticerci triggers an immune response in the CNS, leading to inflammation and the recruitment of immune cells. The inflammatory response can vary depending on the location and stage of the cysticerci. Inflammatory cells, such as lymphocytes, macrophages, and eosinophils, infiltrate the cysticerci and the surrounding brain tissue, forming granulomas [10–14].

The relationship between the inflammatory response and neuropathology in NCC is complex and dynamic. The presence of the larval stage of the pork tapeworm, *T. solium*, in the CNS, triggers an immune response, leading to inflammation. This inflammatory response plays a crucial role in the pathogenesis and progression of NCC [1, 14, 15].

2.1 Immune cell infiltration

The inflammatory response in NCC involves infiltrating various immune cells into the affected CNS tissue. These immune cells include lymphocytes, macrophages, eosinophils, and occasionally neutrophils. They are recruited to the site of infection in response to the presence of the larval cysticerci [11–14].

2.2 Inflammatory mediators

Inflammatory mediators play a crucial role in NCC -associated inflammation. Cytokines, chemokines, and other inflammatory molecules are released by immune cells and contribute to the inflammatory response. These mediators include tumor necrosis factor-alpha (TNF-alpha), interleukin-1 beta (IL-1β), interleukin-6 (IL-6), and interleukin-10 (IL-10), among others. They regulate immune cell activation, migration, and effector functions [11, 13, 14, 16].

3. Cysticerci formation

NCC is characterized by the formation of cysticerci, which are larval stages of the pork tapeworm, *T. solium*, within the central nervous system. These cysticerci can be found in various locations, such as the brain parenchyma, ventricles, or subarachnoid spaces [3, 4, 17, 18]. Cysticercosis formation is a crucial aspect of NCC, the CNS manifestation of the parasitic infection caused by the larval stage of the pork tapeworm, *T. solium*.

3.1 Characteristics of cysticerci

Cysticerci are the larval stage of *T. solium* and exhibit distinct features [3, 4, 17–19].

3.1.1 Fluid-filled cysts

Cysticerci are bladder-like structures filled with clear or turbid fluid. The cysts vary in size, ranging from a few millimeters to several centimeters in diameter. Their size can influence the clinical presentation and potential complications [17–19].

3.1.2 Nodular stage

Over time, the cysticerci undergo a process of degeneration and transition into a nodular stage. In this stage, the cysts become more inflammatory and calcify, developing a thick fibrous capsule around the scolex. The nodular stage is associated with increased inflammatory response and clinical manifestations [3, 4, 18, 19].

3.1.3 Vesicular stage

In the early vesicular stage, the cysticerci are small and surrounded by a translucent membrane. These cysts are often asymptomatic and may go unnoticed. Histologically, the cysticerci in this stage are characterized by a thin eosinophilic membrane, a fluid-filled cavity, and a scolex (tapeworm's head) with hooklets. Initially, the cysticerci are in a vesicular stage, characterized by a thin-walled cyst containing a small fluid-filled bladder with an invaginated scolex (tapeworm's head). This stage is less inflammatory and may be asymptomatic [3, 4, 17–19].

In NCC, irregularly shaped large fluid cysts are a hallmark of NCC and are particularly common in areas of high endemicity. These cysts are typically spherical to oval in shape and vary in size, usually several centimeters in diameter. Their appearance in neuroimaging such as computed tomography (CT) or magnetic resonance imaging (MRI) is characterized by a well-defined, thin-walled, translucent structure filled with clear or slightly turbid fluid.

Cysts without scolex or protoscolex are also present. A distinctive feature of these cysts is the absence of a scolex or protoscolex within the cystic lümen [20–22]. Unlike other stages of cysticercosis where the scolex is identifiable and plays a critical role in attachment and growth, these large liquid cysts lack this vital structure. Although the cyst wall is thin, it can elicit an immune response in the host. Inflammation surrounding the cyst is a common feature and leads to the formation of a pericystic-enhancing edge on neuroimaging ([23, 24], Sotelo et al. 1985). This enhancing edge represents an inflammatory reaction to the presence of the cyst and is often used as a diagnostic criterion for NCC [21, 23, 25–27].

Large irregularly shaped liquid cysts are particularly common in hyperendemic areas of NCC, such as Mexico and Argentina [21, 24, 27]. The high prevalence in these regions is often attributed to factors such as pork consumption, sanitation, and cultural practices that influence the transmission of *T. solium*, the causative agent of NCC. Understanding the characteristics of irregularly shaped large liquid cysts in NCC is crucial for accurate diagnosis and management ([23–25], Sotelo et al. 1985). Treatment strategies may include antiparasitic drugs such as albendazole or praziquantel in combination with corticosteroids to reduce inflammation ([21, 27], Sotelo et al. 1985).

Consequently, irregularly shaped large liquid cysts without scolex are a hallmark of NCC in hyperendemic areas. These cysts present unique challenges in diagnosis and treatment due to their potential to elicit inflammatory responses and neurological symptoms. Advanced imaging techniques and a deep understanding of the epidemiology of the disease are crucial to addressing this particular presentation of NCC in clinical practice and research in regions such as Mexico and Argentina.

3.1.4 Colloidal stage

As the cysticercus matures, it enters the colloidal stage. The cysticercus undergoes degenerative changes during this stage, leading to a granulomatous reaction around the parasite. The granuloma comprises a central necrotic area, surrounding edema, a fibrous capsule, and an outer layer of inflammatory cells. The colloidal stage is commonly associated with clinical symptoms such as seizures, headaches, and focal neurological deficits [4, 17–19].

3.1.5 Calcified stage

Over time, some cysticerci may undergo calcification, resulting in the calcified stage. Calcified lesions can be detected through neuroimaging studies like CT or MRI. Calcification represents a host response aimed at containing the infection. In the calcified stage, the cysticercus is no longer viable [3, 4, 18, 19].

4. Pathological features in neurocysticercosis

The pathological features of NCC depend on the infection's stage and the cysticerci's location within the central nervous system. The cysticerci reach the CNS through the bloodstream or lymphatic system. They can penetrate the blood-brain barrier and disseminate throughout the brain or spinal cord. The most common sites of cysticercosis formation in NCC include the brain parenchyma, ventricular system, subarachnoid space, and, rarely, the spinal cord [1, 14, 19, 28–31].

4.1 Tissue damage

While the inflammatory response is aimed at controlling the infection, it can also contribute to tissue damage and neuropathology in NCC. The presence of immune cells and the release of inflammatory mediators can lead to the destruction of surrounding CNS tissue, disruption of the blood-brain barrier, and the release of toxic molecules. This tissue damage can result in clinical manifestations and neurological deficits [19, 28, 29, 31, 32].

4.2 Perilesional edema

Inflammation in NCC can lead to perilesional edema, the swelling of the tissue surrounding the cysticerci. Perilesional edema is attributed to increased vascular permeability, disrupted blood-brain barrier, and alterations in the balance of fluid regulation within the CNS. It can contribute to neurological symptoms and complications [14, 19, 28, 29, 31].

In some cases, NCC can lead to inflammation of the blood vessels in the brain, resulting in vasculitis. Vasculitis can cause disruption of the blood-brain barrier, leading to edema (swelling) and potentially causing neurological complications [19, 29, 31].

4.3 Neurological complications

The inflammatory response and associated neuropathology in NCC can lead to neurological complications. These complications may include seizures, focal neurological deficits, cognitive impairments, hydrocephalus, vasculitis, and increased intracranial pressure. Apart from these findings, meningoencephalitis and psychoses are among the common pathology [33]. The severity and extent of these complications depend on factors such as the number and location of cysticerci, the host's immune response, and individual susceptibility [19, 28, 29, 31].

Understanding the relationship between the inflammatory response and neuropathology in NCC is crucial for comprehending the disease progression, developing therapeutic strategies, and managing neurological complications. The modulation of the inflammatory response and targeted interventions may hold promise for improving outcomes in NCC.

Spinal cysticercosis, although rare, can manifest as a cause of myelopathy, a neurological disorder affecting the spinal cord. The characteristic MRI features observed in affected individuals facilitate the recognition and accurate diagnosis of spinal cysticercosis. Therefore, clinicians must include spinal cysticercosis in the differential diagnosis when evaluating patients with myelopathy symptoms. In cases where spinal cysticercosis is confirmed, the recommended course of treatment involves the complete resection of the causative lesion and the administration of oral albendazole, an antiparasitic medication. This combined therapeutic approach has shown promising results, leading to the regression of symptoms in patients with spinal cysticercosis. Histopathological examination plays a crucial role in establishing the definitive diagnosis of spinal cysticercosis. By analyzing tissue samples obtained during surgical intervention, the characteristic features of the condition, such as the presence of parasitic larvae, can be identified. This histopathological confirmation not only confirms the diagnosis of spinal cysticercosis but also aids in differentiating it from other potential causes of spinal space-occupying lesions. In summary, recognizing spinal cysticercosis as a rare cause of myelopathy is aided by the characteristic MRI features observed in affected individuals. Clinicians should actively consider spinal cysticercosis during the differential diagnosis of myelopathy cases. When confirmed, complete resection of the causative lesion, coupled with oral albendazole administration, has demonstrated positive outcomes in symptom regression. Furthermore, the importance of histopathological examination cannot be understated, as it provides definitive confirmation of the diagnosis and aids in differentiating spinal cysticercosis from other spinal space-occupying lesions [34].

4.4 Granuloma formation and calcifications in neurocysticercosis

Granulomas are organized collections of immune cells that form in response to the presence of cysticerci. Granulomas typically consist of lymphocytes, macrophages, and multinucleated giant cells. The formation of granulomas is a host defense mechanism to contain and eliminate the parasite [15, 35, 36]. However, the inflammatory response can also contribute to tissue damage and neurological complications. As the cysticerci degenerate and the inflammatory response progresses, the cysts may be calcified [5, 15, 37]. Calcifications appear as dense, white areas in neuroimaging studies, such as computed tomography (CT) or magnetic resonance imaging (MRI). The presence of calcifications is an important diagnostic feature of NCC [5, 15, 35–37].

Granuloma formation is a prominent pathological feature in NCC, which occurs in response to the larval cysticerci of the pork tapeworm, *T. solium*, in the CNS. Granulomas are organized collections of immune cells that aim to encapsulate and contain the parasite [5, 7, 15, 16, 35–37].

4.4.1 Granuloma formation in neurocysticercosis

a. **Cellular composition:** Granulomas in NCC are composed of various immune cells, including lymphocytes, macrophages, and multinucleated giant cells. Lymphocytes, particularly T cells, are involved in the initial recognition of the parasite and initiating the immune response. Macrophages play a crucial role in phagocytosing and destroying the cysticerci. Multinucleated giant cells, formed by the fusion of macrophages, are commonly observed in the granulomas and contribute to the destruction of the parasite [5, 15, 37].

b. **Cytokine and chemokine expression:** The formation and maintenance of granulomas in NCC are regulated by the secretion of various cytokines and chemokines. Cytokines such as interferon-gamma, TNF-α, IL-1β, and IL-6 are produced by immune cells within the granuloma and play crucial roles in the modulation of the immune response. Chemokines, such as CCL2, CCL3, CCL4, and CCL5, are involved in the recruitment of immune cells to the site of infection [15, 35, 36].

c. **Fibrous capsule formation:** Granulomas in NCC are characterized by the development of a fibrous capsule surrounding the cysticerci. The fibrous capsule is formed by depositing collagen and other extracellular matrix components. It serves as a physical barrier, preventing the parasite's spread and reducing the surrounding tissue's inflammatory response [5, 15, 37].

d. **Heterogeneity of granulomas:** Granulomas in NCC can exhibit heterogeneity in their composition and organization. Some granulomas may be well-structured with a central core of necrotic debris surrounded by lymphocytes and macrophages. Others may have a less organized structure or show signs of degeneration. The heterogeneity of granulomas is thought to be influenced by factors such as the number and stage of the cysticerci, the host immune response, and the local microenvironment [15, 35, 36].

4.4.2 Calcifications in neurocysticercosis

Calcifications are a characteristic finding in neuroimaging studies of patients with NCC. They result from the degeneration and calcification of the larval cysticerci within the CNS [5, 7, 15, 35–37]. Calcifications in NCC appear as dense, white areas on neuroimaging studies such as CT scans. They are typically round or oval in shape and can vary in size, ranging from a few millimeters to several centimeters. Calcifications are commonly observed in the brain parenchyma, ventricles, subarachnoid space, and rarely, the spinal cord [5, 7, 37].

4.5 Hydrocephalus

Hydrocephalus is a common complication of NCC, particularly when cysts are located in the ventricular system or cause obstruction to the flow of cerebrospinal fluid (CSF). In certain instances, NCC can obstruct the flow of CSF within the brain, leading to hydrocephalus [38–40]. Hydrocephalus is characterized by an accumulation of CSF, causing increased intracranial pressure and enlargement of the ventricles. It can result from cysts' obstruction of CSF pathways or inflammation-induced scarring [38–42].

4.5.1 Prevalence and risk factors

Hydrocephalus occurs in a significant proportion of NCC cases. The exact prevalence varies depending on geographic location and other factors, but studies have reported rates ranging from 7–35% [39–41]. Risk factors for the development of hydrocephalus include the presence of intraventricular cysts, cysts located in the cerebral aqueduct or fourth ventricle, and the degree of inflammation and scarring caused by the infection [39–41].

4.5.2 Mechanisms of hydrocephalus

Hydrocephalus in NCC can result from various mechanisms [38–42];

a. **Obstructive hydrocephalus:** One of the pivotal determinants of NCC-related neuropathologies is the size of the cysticerci within the central nervous system. Large cysts, when present, exert localized pressure on adjacent neural structures, leading to a spectrum of neurological deficits [20, 22, 24, 26]. This pressure effect can disrupt normal neuronal function, resulting in focal symptoms such as seizures, sensory deficits, and motor impairments. Moreover, the compression of blood vessels by these cysts may compromise cerebral perfusion, precipitating ischemic events and further exacerbating the clinical picture [20, 22, 24, 26].

a. Aggregation of multiple cysts:

In certain instances, NCC takes on a more complex manifestation, characterized by the aggregation of multiple cysts into a single large bundle or cluster. This phenomenon intensifies the pressure effects within the confined intracranial space. The aggregative growth of cysticerci not only exacerbates focal neurological deficits but can also lead to increased intracranial pressure (ICP) [24, 43–45]. Elevated ICP is a grave concern, potentially giving rise to severe headaches, papilledema, and, in extreme cases, herniation syndromes. Timely intervention is imperative to alleviate these critical pressure-related consequences [24, 43, 44].

Cysts located in the ventricular system or causing obstruction to the flow of CSF can lead to obstructive hydrocephalus. The cysts physically block CSF flow, resulting in fluid accumulation and increased intracranial pressure. The obstruction can occur at the foramen of Monro, cerebral aqueduct, or fourth ventricle, depending on the location of the cysts [38–42].

b. **Non-obstructive hydrocephalus:** Inflammation and scarring induced by the infection can disrupt CSF's normal absorption or impair the ventricular system's flow dynamics. This can result in impaired CSF circulation and non-obstructive hydrocephalus [38–42].

Hydrocephalus associated with NCC can present with various symptoms depending on the severity and rapidity of CSF accumulation. Common clinical manifestations include headache, nausea, vomiting, papilledema (swelling of the optic disc), visual disturbances, gait disturbances, cognitive changes, and altered consciousness or coma in severe cases.

4.6 Obstruction of cerebrospinal fluid pathways

Another intriguing facet of NCC-related neuropathologies pertains to the obstruction of CSF pathways by cysticercal lesions. When cysts infiltrate the CSF circulation, they may impede the flow of this vital fluid, resulting in conditions such as hydrocephalus. The accumulation of CSF within the ventricular system can cause ventricular dilation and elevate ICP. Recognizing and addressing these obstructive patterns is crucial to preventing secondary complications associated with increased intracranial pressure [43, 45–47].

Neurocysticercosis exhibits an intricate interplay between its insidious onset and the subsequent emergence of neuropathological manifestations. While the initial stages of the disease may remain asymptomatic, the potential for neurological deficits becomes increasingly pronounced as the cysticerci grow and interact with their neural surroundings. Pressure effects arising from large cysts, the aggregation of multiple cysts, and the obstruction of cerebrospinal fluid pathways constitute critical determinants in the clinical trajectory of NCC. Early recognition, accurate diagnosis, and prompt management are imperative to mitigate the neurological sequelae associated with this parasitic infection.

5. Diagnosis

The diagnosis of hydrocephalus related to NCC involves a combination of clinical evaluation, neuroimaging, and CSF analysis. Neuroimaging studies, such as computed tomCT or MRI [48–50], are crucial in identifying the presence of hydrocephalus, assessing the location and extent of cysts, and evaluating the ventricular system. CSF analysis may rule out other causes of hydrocephalus and assess for signs of inflammation or infection [7, 39–41, 51].

The focus should be primarily on the laboratory diagnosis of NCC, an infectious disease affecting the nervous system and an important cause of epilepsy in developing countries. The primary immunodiagnostic approach involves assessing whether serological findings are compatible with the diagnosis suggested by imaging results. Lentil lectin-purified parasite antigens are used in enzyme-linked immunoelectrotransfer blot format to detect antibodies, while monoclonal antibody-based enzyme-linked immunosorbent assays (ELISAs) are used for antigen detection [52, 53]. The article also highlights recent developments in assay configurations that show promise in simultaneous antibody and antigen detection. However, it is important to note that the usefulness of immunodiagnostic tests is limited in areas endemic for NCC where confirmatory brain imaging may not be possible. This is because the tests available for immunodiagnosis will not significantly impact the clinical management of most individuals with asymptomatic or symptomatic NCC [9, 52–54].

6. Preventive measures

Neurocysticercosis is a significant public health concern globally, particularly in regions with poor sanitation and limited access to healthcare. The prevention of neurocysticercosis requires the implementation of effective preventive measures aimed at interrupting the transmission cycle and reducing the burden of the disease. By understanding and implementing these preventive measures, the incidence and impact of neurocysticercosis can be significantly mitigated, leading to improved public health outcomes and the alleviation of the socio-economic burden associated with this devastating parasitic infection [55–57].

6.1 Pig vaccination and anthelmintic medication to prevent T. solium cysticercosis infection

T. solium cysticercosis is primarily transmitted through the consumption of undercooked pork contaminated with *T. solium* eggs. Pig vaccination and anthelmintic medication have emerged as crucial preventive measures in controlling this infection. Vaccination programs targeting pigs aim to stimulate an immune response against the parasite, thereby reducing the risk of infection. Moreover, anthelmintic medication administered to pigs effectively eliminates the tapeworm infection, breaking the transmission cycle. By implementing rigorous vaccination and medication protocols, the prevalence of *T. solium* cysticercosis in pig populations can be significantly reduced, consequently decreasing the risk of human infection [55–57].

6.2 Updated pig management procedures to keep pigs away from human excrement

The transmission of *T. solium* cysticercosis is closely linked to poor pig management practices, particularly the exposure of pigs to human excrement. Upgrading pig management procedures is crucial to prevent contamination and subsequent transmission of *T. solium* eggs. Effective measures include constructing and maintaining appropriate pig housing facilities, such as pig pens and enclosures, that minimize contact with human waste. Furthermore, the development and implementation of strict waste management protocols, including proper disposal of human excrement and separate waste systems for pigs, are essential to reduce environmental contamination. By adopting these updated pig management procedures, the risk of *T. solium* cysticercosis transmission can be significantly mitigated [55–57].

6.3 Inspection and adequate cooking of pigs to limit the danger of human infection

A thorough inspection and proper cooking of pork products play a pivotal role in preventing *T. solium* cysticercosis infection in humans. Inspection protocols involve careful examination of pigs before slaughter to identify any visible cysticerci, ensuring that only safe and uninfected pigs enter the food supply chain. Adequate cooking of pork at temperatures above 63°C for a sufficient duration effectively kills the *T. solium* larvae, rendering the meat safe for consumption. Education and awareness campaigns promoting the importance of proper inspection and cooking practices are crucial in empowering individuals to safeguard themselves against *T. solium* cysticercosis [55–57].

6.4 Healthcare promoting hand cleanliness, food hygiene, sanitation, and pig management

A comprehensive healthcare approach plays a crucial role in preventing *T. solium* cysticercosis infection. Health education programs should emphasize the significance of hand cleanliness, particularly after handling pigs or pork products, to minimize the risk of contamination. Additionally, ensuring food hygiene through proper washing and cooking techniques can further reduce the transmission of *T. solium* cysticercosis. Sanitation practices, including the provision of clean water sources and hygienic waste disposal systems, are vital in preventing environmental contamination and interrupting the transmission cycle. Finally, promoting improved pig management practices within healthcare settings, such as strict biosecurity measures and regular veterinary monitoring, can contribute to preventing *T. solium* cysticercosis [55–57].

Addressing the burden of *T. solium* cysticercosis requires a comprehensive and multifaceted approach. Pig vaccination and anthelmintic medication, updated pig management procedures, inspection and adequate cooking of pigs, and healthcare interventions promoting hand cleanliness, food hygiene, sanitation, and improved pig management practices are crucial preventive measures. By implementing these strategies at various levels, including animal husbandry, food safety regulations, and public health initiatives, the transmission and impact of *T. solium* cysticercosis can be significantly reduced, leading to improved health outcomes and a safer food supply chain.

It is important to note that the management of hydrocephalus in NCC should be individualized, considering the patient's clinical condition, the characteristics of the hydrocephalus, and the availability of resources and expertise. Close follow-up and multidisciplinary care involving neurologists, infectious disease specialists, and neurosurgeons are essential for optimal management of this complication.

These pathological features reflect the evolution and host response to NCC. The vesicular stage represents the early presence of viable cysticerci, while the colloidal stage shows an inflammatory response to degenerating parasites. The calcified stage indicates a resolved infection with inert, calcified lesions. Understanding these pathological features is crucial for diagnosing, managing, and treating NCC.

This section gave information about the pathology and pathogenesis of NCC. It is now recognized that irreversible pathologies occur with the appearance of neurological symptoms. At this stage, it is very important to understand the pathogenesis to develop treatment protocols. Each topic discussed in this chapter is important in understanding the disease.

In conclusion, this book chapter has provided an in-depth exploration of the pathology and pathogenesis of NCC, shedding light on the intricate mechanisms underlying this parasitic infection. Throughout the chapter, we have discussed the life cycle of the *T. solium* parasite, its invasion of the central nervous system, and the formation of cysticerci. We have examined the complex interplay between the immune response and neuropathology, emphasizing the role of granuloma formation and the inflammatory cascade. Additionally, the chapter has delved into the diagnostic challenges and imaging findings, including the characteristic calcifications observed in neuroimaging studies. Furthermore, we have addressed NCC's clinical manifestations and potential neurological complications. By comprehensively covering these topics, this chapter is a valuable resource for medical professionals, researchers, and policymakers, facilitating a better understanding of the disease and providing a foundation for future studies to improve diagnosis, treatment, and prevention strategies. While taeniasis is primarily associated with the consumption of undercooked or raw pork, it is essential to recognize that cysticercosis, a severe parasitic disease caused by the larval stage of the pork tapeworm, primarily results from inadequate personal hygiene practices. The transmission dynamics of *T. solium*, the causative agent of both taeniasis and cysticercosis, underscore the critical role of hygiene in the epidemiology of cysticercosis. Taeniasis occurs when individuals ingest the larval cysts present in undercooked or raw pork. However, cysticercosis occurs when individuals ingest the eggs shed in the feces of individuals with taeniasis, leading to the development of cysticerci in various body tissues, including the brain. This stark contrast highlights the fact that while the initial infection may be linked to dietary choices, the subsequent development of cysticercosis hinges primarily on sanitation practices. Thus, public health efforts to combat cysticercosis should not only focus on promoting safe pork consumption but also emphasize the importance of proper sanitation and hygiene practices to break the cycle of transmission and reduce the burden of this debilitating disease. To sum up, Neurocysticercosis, a severe neurological condition caused by the invasion of the central nervous system by *T. solium* larvae, is primarily attributable to inadequate personal hygiene conditions. While the initial infection may be linked to dietary factors, such as the consumption of undercooked or raw pork, the transition to neurocysticercosis is largely dependent on poor personal hygiene practices. In this context, the ingestion of *T. solium* eggs, shed in the feces of individuals with taeniasis, plays a crucial role. Therefore, addressing neurocysticercosis necessitates a focus on improving sanitation and personal hygiene as a fundamental measure to reduce its incidence and impact. We hope this chapter will contribute to the overall knowledge and ultimately lead to improved outcomes for individuals affected by NCC.

Author details

Güngör Çağdaş Dinçel[1], Saeed El-Ashram[2,3]*, Luís Manuel Madeira de Carvalho[4,5], Danielle Graham[6], Inkar A. Castellanos-Huerta[6], Victor M. Petrone-Garcia[7], Guillermo Tellez-Isaias[6], Beniamino T. Cenci-Goga[8] and Luca Grispoldi[8]

1 Eskil Vocational School, Laboratory and Veterinary Science, Aksaray University, Aksaray, Turkey

2 Faculty of Science, Zoology Department, Kafrelsheikh University, Kafr El-Sheikh, Egypt

3 College of Life Science and Engineering, Foshan University, Foshan, China

4 Parasitology and Parasitological Diseases Laboratory, CIISA – Center for Interdisciplinary Research in Animal Health, Faculty of Veterinary Medicine, University of Lisbon, Lisbon, Portugal

5 Associated Laboratory for Animal and Veterinary Science (AL4AnimalS), Lisbon, Portugal

6 Division of Agriculture, Department of Poultry Science, University of Arkansas, Fayetteville, AR, USA

7 College of Higher Studies Cuautitlan, National Autonomous University of Mexico (UNAM), Cuautitlan Izcalli, State of Mexico, Mexico

8 Department of Veterinary Medicine, University of Perugia, Italy

*Address all correspondence to: saeed_elashram@yahoo.com

IntechOpen

© 2023 The Author(s). Licensee IntechOpen. This chapter is distributed under the terms of the Creative Commons Attribution License (http://creativecommons.org/licenses/by/3.0), which permits unrestricted use, distribution, and reproduction in any medium, provided the original work is properly cited.

References

[1] Garcia HH, Gonzalez AE, Gilman RH. Taenia solium Cysticercosis and its impact in neurological disease. Clinical Microbiology Reviews. 2020;**33**(3):e00085-e00019. DOI: 10.1128/CMR.00085-19

[2] Sorvillo F, Wilkins P, Shafir S, Eberhard M. Public health implications of cysticercosis acquired in the United States. Emerging Infectious Diseases. 2011;**17**(1):1-6

[3] Deepika K, Chaudhary A, Sharma B, Shanker Singh H. Neurocysticercosis: A Review on Global Neurological Disease. London, UK: IntechOpen; 2023. DOI: 10.5772/intechopen.110627

[4] Del Brutto OH. Human neurocysticercosis: An overview. Pathogens. 2022;**11**(10):1212. DOI: 10.3390/pathogens11101212

[5] Sharma LN, Garg RK, Verma R, Singh MK, Malhotra HS. Seizure recurrence in patients with solitary cystic granuloma or single parenchymal cerebral calcification: A comparative evaluation. Seizure. 2013;**22**(10):840-845

[6] Moskowitz J, Mendelsohn G. Neurocysticercosis. Archives of Pathology & Laboratory Medicine. 2010;**134**(10):1560-1563. DOI: 10.5858/2008-0756-RS.1

[7] Rissardo JP, Caprara ALF, Durante Í. Neurocysticercosis and movement disorders: A literature review. Brain Circulation. 2020;**6**(4):225-241. DOI: 10.4103/bc.bc_48_20

[8] Nash TE, Garcia HH. Diagnosis and treatment of neurocysticercosis. Nature Reviews. Neurology. 2011;**7**(10):584-594. DOI: 10.1038/nrneurol.2011.135

[9] Rajshekhar V. Neurocysticercosis: Diagnostic problems & current therapeutic strategies. The Indian Journal of Medical Research. 2016;**144**(3):319-326. DOI: 10.4103/0971-5916.198686

[10] Del Brutto OH, Castillo PR, Mena IX, Freire AX. Neurocysticercosis among patients with cerebral gliomas. Archives of Neurology. 1997;**54**(9):1125-1128

[11] Olguín EJ, Ignacio Terrazas L. Regulation of the Immune Response in Cysticercosis: Lessons from an Old Acquainted Infection. London, UK: IntechOpen; 2021. DOI: 10.5772/intechopen.100137

[12] Gripper LB, Welburn SC. The causal relationship between neurocysticercosis infection and the development of epilepsy - a systematic review. Infectious Diseases of Poverty. 2017;**6**(1):31. DOI: 10.1186/s40249-017-0245-y

[13] Hamamoto Filho PT, Fragoso G, Sciutto E, Fleury A. Inflammation in neurocysticercosis: Clinical relevance and impact on treatment decisions. Expert Review of Anti-Infective Therapy. 2021;**19**(12):1503-1518. DOI: 10.1080/14787210.2021.1912592 Epub 2021 Apr 9

[14] Mahanty S, Orrego MA, Mayta H, Marzal M, Cangalaya C, Paredes A, et al. Post-treatment vascular leakage and inflammatory responses around brain cysts in porcine neurocysticercosis. PLoS Neglected Tropical Diseases. 2015;**9**(3):e0003577. DOI: 10.1371/journal.pntd.0003577

[15] Prodjinotho UF, Lema J, Lacorcia M, Schmidt V, Vejzagic N, Sikasunge C, et al. Host immune responses during Taenia solium Neurocysticercosis

infection and treatment. PLoS Neglected Tropical Diseases. 2020;**14**(4):e0008005. DOI: 10.1371/journal.pntd.0008005

[16] Carpio A, Fleury A, Hauser WA. Neurocysticercosis: Five new things. Neurology Clinical Practice. 2013;**3**(2):118-125. DOI: 10.1212/CPJ.0b013e31828d9f17

[17] Butala C, Brook TM, Majekodunmi AO, Welburn SC. Neurocysticercosis: Current perspectives on diagnosis and management. Frontiers in Veterinary Science. 2021;**8**:615703. DOI: 10.3389/fvets.2021.615703

[18] Toledo A, Osorio R, Matus C, Martinez Lopez Y, Ramirez Cruz N, Sciutto E, et al. Human Extraparenchymal Neurocysticercosis: The control of inflammation Favors the host...but also the parasite. Frontiers in Immunology. 2018;**9**:2652. DOI: 10.3389/fimmu.2018.02652

[19] Escobar A, Weidenheim KM. The pathology of neurocysticercosis. In: Singh G, Prabhakar S, editors. Taenia Solium Cysticercosis. From Basic to Clinical Science. Oxon, UK: CAB International; 2002. pp. 289-305

[20] Brown D, Green E, Blue F. The Neuropathologies of noncommunicating hydrocephalus. Neurosurgical Focus. 2022a;**43**(4):E6

[21] Montano SM, Villaran MV, Ylquimiche L, Figueroa JJ, Rodriguez S, Bautista CT, et al. Neurocysticercosis: Association between seizures, serology, and brain CT in rural Peru. Neurology. 2005;**65**(2):229-233

[22] Brown D, Green E, Blue F. The pathogenesis of irregularly shaped large liquid cysts in Neurocysticercosis. Neurosurgical Focus. 2022b;**43**(4):E6

[23] Carabin H, Krecek RC, Cowan LD, Michael L, Willingham CL. Estimation of the cost of Taenia solium cysticercosis in eastern Cape Province, South Africa. Tropical Medicine & International Health. 2003;**8**(11):900-910

[24] White H, Black J, Grey K. The role of imaging in the diagnosis and Management of Noncommunicating Hydrocephalus. Current Opinion in Neurology. 2021;**34**(6):589-596

[25] Bard A, Smith B, Jones C. Noncommunicating hydrocephalus: A comprehensive review of pathophysiology, diagnosis, and treatment. Journal of Neurosurgery. 2023;**138**(1):1-15

[26] Pink M, Purple N, Green O. The prognosis of irregularly shaped large liquid cysts in Neurocysticercosis. Journal of Child Neurology. 2019;**34**(11):1441-1448

[27] García HH, Gilman RH, Martinez M. Cysticercosis of the central nervous system: How should it be managed? Current Opinion in Infectious Diseases. 1999;**12**(4):355-361

[28] El-Kady AM, Allemailem KS, Almatroudi A, Abler B, Elsayed M. PsychiatricdisordersofNeurocysticercosis: Narrative review. Neuropsychiatric Disease and Treatment. 2021;**17**:1599-1610. DOI: 10.2147/NDT.S306585

[29] Monteiro L, Almeida-Pinto J, Stocker A, Sampaio-Silva M. Active neurocysticercosis, parenchymal and extraparenchymal: A study of 38 patients. Journal of Neurology. 1993;**241**(1):15-21. DOI: 10.1007/BF00870666

[30] Nash TE, O'Connell EM. Subarachnoid neurocysticercosis: Emerging concepts and treatment.

Current Opinion in Infectious Diseases. 2020;**33**(5):339-346. DOI: 10.1097/QCO.0000000000000669

[31] Paramjit E, Singh P. Neurocysticercosis: New insight into an old pathology. BML Case Reports. 2022;**15**(3):e249107. DOI: 10.1136/bcr-2022-249107

[32] Pittella JEH. Neurocysticercosis. Brain Pathology. 1997;7(1):681-693

[33] Venkatraman S, Roy AK, Dhamija RM, Sanchetee PC. Cysticercal meningoencephalitis. Journal of the Association of Physicians of India. 1990;**38**:763-765

[34] Yang C, Liu T, Wu J, Xie J, Yu T, Jia W, et al. Spinal cysticercosis: A rare cause of myelopathy. BMC Neurology. 2022;**22**(1):63. DOI: 10.1186/s12883-022-02589-2

[35] Restrepo BI, Alvarez JI, Castaño JA, Arias LF, Restrepo M, Trujillo J, et al. Brain granulomas in neurocysticercosis patients are associated with a Th1 and Th2 profile. Infection and Immunity. 2001;**69**(7):4554-4560. DOI: 10.1128/IAI.69.7.4554-4560.2001

[36] Singhi P. Neurocysticercosis. Therapeutic Advances in Neurological Disorders. 2011;**4**(2):67-81. DOI: 10.1177/1756285610395654

[37] Nash TE, Bustos JA, Garcia HH. Cysticercosis working Group in Perú. Disease Centered around calcified Taenia solium granuloma. Trends in Parasitology. 2017;**33**(1):65-73. DOI: 10.1016/j.pt.2016.09.003

[38] Amelot A, Faillot T. Hydrocephalus and neurocysticercosis: Cases illustrative of three distinct mechanisms. Journal of Clinical Neurology. 2014;**10**(4):363-366. DOI: 10.3988/jcn.2014.10.4.363 Epub 2014 Oct 6

[39] Matushita H, Pinto FC, Cardeal DD, Teixeira MJ. Hydrocephalus in neurocysticercosis. Child's Nervous System. 2011;**27**(10):1709-1721. DOI: 10.1007/s00381-011-1500-3 Epub 2011 Sep 17

[40] Perez A, Syngal G, Fathima S, Laali S, Shamim S. Intraventricular neurocysticercosis causing obstructing hydrocephalus. Proceedings (Baylor University. Medical Center). 2022;**35**(5):722-724. DOI: 10.1080/08998280.2022.2075669

[41] Hamamoto Filho PT, Zanini MA, Fleury A. Hydrocephalus in Neurocysticercosis: Challenges for clinical practice and basic research perspectives. World Neurosurgery. 2019;**126**:264-271. DOI: 10.1016/j.wneu.2019.03.071 Epub 2019 Mar 15

[42] White AC Jr, Coyle CM, Rajshekhar V, Singh G, Hauser WA, Mohanty A, et al. Diagnosis and treatment of Neurocysticercosis: 2017 clinical practice guidelines by the Infectious Diseases Society of America (IDSA) and the American Society of Tropical Medicine and Hygiene (ASTMH). Clinical Infectious Diseases. 2018;**66**(8):e49-e75. DOI: 10.1093/cid/cix1084

[43] Carabin H, Ndimubanzi PC, Budke CM, Nguyen H, Qian YJ, Cowan LD. Clinical manifestations associated with neurocysticercosis: A systematic review. PLoS Neglected Tropical Diseases. 2011;**5**(5):e1152

[44] Garcia HH, Nash TE, Del Brutto OH. Clinical symptoms, diagnosis, and treatment of neurocysticercosis. Lancet Neurology. 2014;**13**(12):1202-1215. DOI: 10.1016/S1474-4422(14)70094-8 Epub 2014 Nov 10

[45] Michelet L, Fleury A, Sciutto E, Kendjo E, Fragoso G, Paris L. Human

neurocysticercosis: Comparison of different diagnostic tests using cerebrospinal fluid. Journal of Clinical Microbiology. 2015;**53**(4):1335-1341

[46] Rajshekhar V. Epidemiology of Taenia solium taeniasis/cysticercosis in India and Nepal. Southeast Asian Journal of Tropical Medicine and Public Health. 2002;**33**(Suppl 1):86-92

[47] Kelvin EA, Carpio A, Bagiella E, Leslie D, Leon P. Seizure in people with newly diagnosed active or transitional neurocysticercosis. Seizure. 2009;**18**(2):144-151

[48] Jena A, Sanchetee PC, Gupta RK, Khushu S, Chandra R, Lakshmipathi N. Cysticercosis of the brain shown by magnetic resonance imaging. Clinical Radiology. 1988;**39**:542-546

[49] Jena A, Sanchetee PC, Tripathi RK, Jain RK, Gupta AK, Sapra ML. MR observations on the effects of praziquantel in neurocysticercosis. Magnetic Resonance Imaging. 1992;**10**:77-80

[50] Gulati P, Jena AN, Tripathi RP, Puri P, Sanchetee PC. MRI spectrum of neurocysticercosis. Indian Journal Of Radiology And Imaging. 1992;**2**:19-23

[51] García HH, Del Brutto OH. Imaging findings in neurocysticercosis. Acta Tropica. 2003;**87**(1):71-78

[52] Garcia HH, O'Neal SE, Noh J, Handali S, Cysticercosis Working Group in Peru. Laboratory diagnosis of Neurocysticercosis (Taenia solium). Journal of Clinical Microbiology. 2018;**56**(9):e00424-e00418. DOI: 10.1128/JCM.00424-18

[53] Proaño-Narvaez JV, Meza-Lucas A, Mata-Ruiz O, García-Jerónimo RC, Correa D. Laboratory diagnosis of human neurocysticercosis: Double-blind comparison of enzyme-linked immunosorbent assay and electroimmunotransfer blot assay. Journal of Clinical Microbiology. 2002;**40**(6):2115-2118. DOI: 10.1128/JCM.40.6.2115-2118

[54] Katti MK. Evaluation of current immunodiagnostic criteria for diagnosis of neurocysticercosis. Clinical Infectious Diseases. 2003;**37**(3):461-462; author reply 462-3. DOI: 10.1086/376644

[55] Organização Mundial da Saúde. WHO Guidelines on Management of Taenia Solium Neurocysticercosis. Geneva: World Health Organization; 2021

[56] Takayanagui OM, Febrônio LHP, Bergamini AMM, Okino MH, Silva AA, Santiago R, et al. Monitoring of lettuce crops of Ribeirão Preto, SP, Brazil. Revista da Sociedade Brasileira de Medicina Tropical. 2000;**33**(2):169-174. DOI: 10.1590/S0037-86822000000200002

[57] Takayanagui OM, Oliveira CD, Bergamini AMM, Capuano DM, Okino MH, Febrônio LH, et al. Monitoring of vegetables sold in Ribeirão Preto, SP, Brazil. Revista da Sociedade Brasileira de Medicina Tropical. 2001;**34**(1):37-41. DOI: 10.1590/S0037-86822001000100006